"This writer speaks about day to day events that happen in hospitals everywhere; she does so with great insight, wit and compassion. She also shows her admiration for the fortitude of her patients. Although there is pain and heartache there is also happy outcomes too. Read this book and expect to shed tears of both sadness and laughter."
Bill Brady,
Columnist, The London Free Press

"This book contains a collection of short stories from the authors many years in nursing. They are told with compassion, sensitivity and often humour. This former nurse never forgets her own humanity or that of her patients while providing them with the care they need."
L. June Stevenson,
Editor, Glad Tidings

"From the other side of the Bed," is a book of short anecdotes about the trials and tribulations encountered by someone in the medical profession. Victoria's stories are at the same time funny, sad, enriching and thought provoking. After reading this book one realizes that almost certainly we ourselves will one day be the person, "Inside," the bed that she speaks about!"
Edward G. Janzen.
Editor, Publisher, Canadian Stories Magazine

"From the other side of the Bed," is a collection of sensitively written experiences in the life of a hospital nurse. Some of the stories are downright funny, others may evoke a tear or two, but all of them will prove enlightening."
Eileen Cade-Edwards, Author

"In her first book this writer gives readers an amusing, at times heartbreaking, as well as hilarious view of life as a nurse in the 1970's. This is a delightful read as it takes you into the very heart of the nursing profession. It leaves you with a resounding appreciation for the special women and men who work there."
Roberta McClelland,
Oxford Book Shop

"Victoria Stirling has given a new perspective to the nursing profession in her book. The inspirations behind her stories are the people that she met during her long nursing career."
Jen Mayville,
South London, The Reporter

"With a warm and compassionate approach Victoria Stirling views the troubles and foibles of her patients. Her book will give you an insight into what it takes to be a nurse."
Ruth Zavitz, Writer

"Victoria's book allows us to put ourselves in the shoes of a professional nurse, and to study and share in the various situations that comprise its many tales. Though unannounced, and perhaps unintentional I found that many of the stories contained a lesson, a moral to the story. I suggest that you read one chapter a day as a form of relaxation and reflection. Life will eventually see all of us in an uncomfortable medical situation and this book delivers exactly what it promises, tales "From the other side of the Bed."
Mark Moran,
Publisher, Daytripping Magazine

"Victoria's book has an apt title, "From the other side of the bed." It's mainly from that vantagepoint that a nurse makes contact with patients.
Her stories are down to earth and tell of real life experiences, and they are all easily understood.
I found this book to be a most enjoyable read."
Gladys Nolan, Author

Victoria
Stirling

FROM THE OTHER
SIDE
OF THE BED

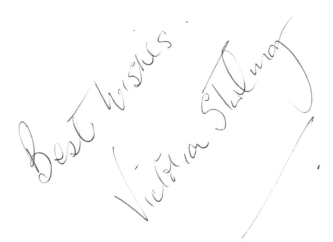

Best wishes

Victoria Stirling

Published by
Stirling Publishing
London, Ontario
Canada

Original artwork/copyright 2001.
Artist, Frank Northgrave.
London, Ontario

Earlier versions of some of these stories appeared in The Annals of St. Anne de Beaupre. Messenger of the Sacred Heart, Glad Tidings, Pioneer News, Canadian Stories and The Daytripper.

Copyright c 2001, Victoria Stirling
Manufactured and printed in Canada

National Library of Canada Cataloging in Publication Data.
1. Stirling, Victoria, 1933- 2. Nurses--Canada--Biography
1. From the other side of the bed

RT37.S76A3 2001   610.73'092   C2001-903789-9

ISBN # 0-9689894-0-3

For the Special People in my life

To my husband Harvey, for all his love and ceaseless encouragement; thank you!

And, Anne, our daughter, who first nudged me into starting this project, and tirelessly taught me how to use a computer; who also arranged my stories into a book format.

I'm grateful also to Richard, our grandson, who never doubted that I would succeed, and Andrew, our son, for his unflagging confidence in me.

Acknowledgements

Thanks to all those people who supported me throughout this project.

Much indebtedness to my friends in the Professional Writer's Workshop group, your expertise in reviewing steered me in the right direction. To Ruth Zavitz, your assistance and helpful suggestions made that difficult task of rewriting much easier.

My endless gratitude goes also to Edward Janzen, the Editor of Canadian Stories. He read many of my stories and assisted with the editing.

CONTENTS

Introduction

I'm an absolute coward when it comes to being pierced with sharp objects and the sight of blood can make me ill; yet I chose to become a nurse. How come?

Like thousands of other women and I'm sure some men as well it happened because of a strong desire to want to help others. Perhaps, in my own case it was related to an over-powering maternal instinct.

Whatever it was that drew me into this profession it is something that I would not have missed doing. It's a field of work that gives the practitioner many non-monetary rewards. One gets personal satisfaction from knowing that you have been able to assist other human beings when they are most vulnerable.

My entry into this profession started in 1973 when I responded to an advertisement in the local paper for nurse's aides. The dormant feelings I'd had for years about nursing were prompted into action. Life up to that point had been too busy. Now with my family well on the way to being self-sufficient it was my time to look at doing something outside of the home.

With some trepidation, I submitted my application not really knowing what was expected. There followed an intensive interview and I was hired to work in a chronic care facility. From that humble start I went on to become a Registered Nursing Assistant, and almost completed the two-year program to become a Registered Nurse.

It was my privilege during my years of practice to work in many different areas. I was also afforded the marvelous opportunity to represent my peers for three years on the governing body for nursing, The College of Nurses of Ontario.

However, this book is not about me. It's about some of the many, unforgettable people that I've worked with or had as patients. Its time to let some of their stories be told and shared.

Because it is important to maintain the anonymity of people, names of people and places have been omitted or changed. Also as with all memoirs I've taken some artistic license with the dialogue. Nonetheless, this in no way alters the reality of the experiences recorded here.

Foreword

My mother is someone who, as a child, lived through the London Blitz. After the war, she joined the Royal Navy where she met, fell in love and married my father, who was a Royal Navy seaman.

Within two years, she had me and then fours years later my brother. Like most women of that time, she was a stay-at-home mum. Our family at first lived in a small flat in my father's hometown of Dundee, Scotland. My father was away from home a lot on foreign commissions, some taking years. One of my favorite stories is that for the first few years of my life I traveled with my mother on hundreds of train rides to visit her family in London. No wonder I have had the wanderlust for many years!

When my brother and I were still children, our family went with my father to his posting in Malta. I will never forget that experience. Christmas dinner on the beach and the many ethnic sights I witnessed on this Orthodox Catholic Island. I also remember my mother choosing to live amongst the Maltese people rather than in the exclusive English area. I played with Maltese children and this is what I am sure influenced my belief that people everywhere are the same.

Then it came time for my father to retire and the decision was made to immigrate. New Zealand was the first choice but due to the shipyard strikes, Canada became the destination. I remember clearly my mother looking down from the plane on her new home, London and exclaiming, "Where are all the houses?" We had chosen the Forest City and at that, time there were so many trees the town was nearly invisible from the air.

My mother worked retail and then in her forties decided to train to be a nurse, something she had always dreamed of being as a girl. Today no-one bats an eye at changing careers in mid-life. However, in those days it was unusual and made my mother a pioneer and a role model for me.

The reason my mother credits me for nudging her to write this book is understated. After a surgery that went very badly, I was very ill and needed one on one care. Usually, I would not stand for unnecessary coddling, but with my mother's patient and gentle care in tending to my basic human needs, I saw firsthand the care she had given each of her patients. I, like them, maintained a dignity and felt completely at ease with her ministering. Applying the many dressings to a horribly infected wound or giving a sponge bath that she knew would make me feel better, I saw in her the quintessential nurse. My mother was Florence Nightingale and all she embodied.

As I recovered, I remembered my mother's stories and this combined with her love of writing, I not only nudged, I pushed her to the job. I told her that her experiences could be her legacy to a profession where her manner of nursing is, what I believe, is a calling. I am very proud of her. I hope you the reader will enjoy the stories and in them see the depth of her caring.

Anne Stirling
November 2001

An Innocent Remark

Mr. Noble was an elderly gentleman who loved to talk about his former home. Since I had come to Canada myself from England, I sympathized with some of his loneliness. He did not get many outside visitors. Whenever he was assigned to me I'd encourage him to reminiscence and speak about his times past.

His round, full face would always light up when he recalled living in Holland. The memories he had of field after field of tulips of every kind and color gave him a great deal of pleasure. "You could not see anything else, when they were all in bloom, "he would tell me repeatedly.

He had been raised and worked his early years on a farm. He delighted in seeing my reaction when he remembered, and told me, "How good the warm milk tasted when it had just come straight from the cow." The grimace that I always made would get a loud bellow of laughter every time from him.

He would also remind me of how many people in his country rode bikes compared to the few here in Canada. "Is better to ride on two wheels than always inside one with four. Is healthier too." I would just smile and nod at his comments.

Because of a heavier assignment load in the chronic care facility where I worked, and Mr. Noble was a patient, giving him, this extra time to chat was not always an option. The barest essential care was all I could provide. This would upset him and he would become downcast and sad. When he got like that there wasn't much a person could do to cheer him up

In this institution, there were people of all ages and in a wide range of health disorders. The staff was usually so busy filling the physical needs of our patients that we had little time to concern ourselves about our client's mental well being. Still, it bothered me greatly to see this old gentleman so dejected.

He was confined to a wheelchair, because of his inability to stand or walk, so this as well limited his activities. I made the suggestion that he might like to be taken outside for awhile, but that didn't get any positive response from him. Since I had other patients to feed and dress, I had to leave Mr. Noble sitting in his chair gazing pensively out of his window. I promised to return as quickly as possible. As I made my way out the door, I murmured, "Just try to keep your pecker up."

The immediate reaction from him startled me. He started to laugh so loud and so much, he went into a major coughing fit. Looking into his reddened, perspiring face I didn't know what to think.

The Head-Nurse hearing all the commotion tore down the hall into Mr. Noble's room. Although he was beginning to calm down a little, it was still puzzling me why he had reacted so violently. When we finally were able to get his coughing and laughter under control Mr. Noble said, "Of course I knew what you meant nurse, but it wasn't something that I had expected to hear."

He pulled out a handkerchief and wiped his face. Grinning at us both, he added, "Here in this part of the world that has a totally different meaning, and it is in no way related to a persons chin."

When he told me the North American definition, I was mortified. I was also able to understand why he had behaved the way that he had.

The dressing down that followed from my supervisor did not help me feel any better. She scathingly said, "that it was very important to use care when talking with elderly patients because of their frail state. I hardly think that you would want to be the cause of someone's sudden demise."

Of course, I did not want that to happen and told her so. I left her office feeling I'd done something terrible.

Mr. Noble needed to be checked again so I walked back into his room. But, instead of a despondent, unhappy man I found him sitting straight up in his chair humming a merry tune. His round face beamed, and he saucily winked.

The change in him was great to see. After that incident, Mr. Noble always had a special smile and a chuckle when I provided him with his care. It amazed me how something said so innocently was able to brighten up someone else's life so much.

From then on, however, before verbalizing anymore of my old English adages I made certain I knew the correct definition. One faux pas, as this one, was quite enough for me.

Tears Aren't Always Bad

"Oh! No, " I loudly exclaimed. "What's up with Mrs. Richie?"
Jean the other nurse on duty looked up from her charting.
"Could be that she's found out what her diagnosis is, " she said.

"I didn't know that her results were back yet, " I replied.

"Well, I believe the medical team went in today to see her, "
Jean nodded her head at me. "So they must know something."

Mrs. Richie was a middle-aged, married lady. She had
arrived on the ward to undergo some tests because she had
been having some unexplained abdominal pain.

"But, "as she told me when I'd admitted her, "I'm sure that
it's nothing. I've just got a lazy bowel that's all."

I smiled at her self-diagnosis, which is a bad habit of many
people. "Let's hope and pray that that's all it is, "I said.

Mrs. Richie gave a deep chuckle. "Nurse, " she said, "
praying is something I consider myself to be an expert at. How
about you? Do you pray at all?"

"Yes, "I admitted, "I pray a lot. I find it helps me cope a bit
better with whatever happens in the day. "

"You've got that right nurse, "Mrs.Richie said. "I know I will
be doing a lot of it while I am here. As well as reading more of
my Bible."

"Well, "I told her, "If you like I'll give your name to my
prayer group. We meet once a week for prayers and Bible
study."

"You'd do that for me?" Mrs. Richie sounded surprised.

I nodded, "Of course I would. Isn't that what we are
supposed to do for each other?"

She inclined her head, "Yes, but you're busy helping people
in so many other ways why would you want to be bothered
doing that for me."

I touched her Bible which she had laid on the overbed table. "It's all in there even if we don't always follow what it says, and some days it's harder than other days to do everything."

Mrs. Richie smiled and wagged a finger at me. "It's important though that we never tire of trying."

After I had had this conversation with this patient, she would on occasion tell me that she also said a prayer for me. I'd thank her for her thoughtfulness.

This lady underwent several tests for her stomach disorder. Although a couple of them were not pleasant to experience, she took them all in her stride and never complained.

Now here she was talking, and sobbing on the telephone. I had to find out what was causing her so much anguish.

Going over to the public pay phone, I gave a little wave. She didn't acknowledge that she had seen me coming. As I didn't want to alarm her by appearing suddenly by her side I noisily rattled some keys. She looked up at me with tears still streaming down her face.

"Mrs.Richie, " I gently said. "Whatever is the matter?"

She gulped and let out a heart-wrenching sigh. "Oh nurse. The doctors have just given me the results of all those awful tests I had."

I placed an arm around her shoulders. "Mrs.Richie, "What did they tell you?"

She took a moment to speak to the person on the other end of the telephone. Her tears had subsided but she still took in large gulps of air as a way of catching her breath.

I offered her several Kleenex. "Here, it might help if you give your nose a blow." I said.

She did as I suggested once she had finished her call; she placed her hands on my shoulders. As I looked into this woman's tear-stained face I could only suspect the worst had happened. Her diagnosis must have been for something terminal.

Mrs.Richie smiled at me. "Oh! Nurse, nurse, nurse." she murmured, "This has been a most unusual day."

"In what way?" I asked.

Her blue eyes again filled with tears. "It's nothing. I have got nothing wrong. "She said. "All it is, is an irritable bowel. Some medication and a change of diet will soon fix it up."

Then I realized why she had been crying. It wasn't because of any bad news; it was over the relief that she'd felt that it wasn't anything serious. I had been far too hasty and had jumped to all the wrong conclusions.

"Oh! Mrs.Richie, " I said, giving her a squeeze. "I am very pleased for you. Smiling, she patted my back. "Believe me, you can't be nowhere near as happy as I am right now."

I am sure that she was right. We turned and arm in arm happily walked back to her room.

The New Dad's Dilemma

My favorite area of nursing while in training was the delivery room. There is constantly an element of excitement and anticipation there that I was never able to feel on any other ward. I found it was even more intense when the new parents-to-be were young.

Some fathers welcome the opportunity to be present when the actual birth takes place but this is not always the best plan. Simulating a baby's birth in a classroom does not really prepare some parents for what actually occurs.

John and Eileen Gibbs were expecting their first baby. They arrived on the unit with Eileen wheeled in by a porter and John laden down with a great deal of luggage. When asked why he was carrying so much, John went into a long drawn out explanation.

"My wife wants all this stuff with her, because we've always had it with us during the practice sessions."

"Okay," I said, as I took hold of the two large teddy bears,"I'm just not sure what part these are going to play in the birth of your baby, but if you follow me I'll get your wife admitted.

At the time that I was assigned to this unit, the patients were placed in a small room until they were ready to deliver. This was where I took this couple.

John raised his eyebrows and muttered. "Hmm! It's a bit cramped in here don't you think?'

I had helped his wife out of the wheelchair and she was now sitting on the bed. Her young face grimaced with pain as she held onto her swollen abdomen.

"Oh! For goodness sake," she glared at her husband."Who cares? I certainly don't," she moaned.

"It's all right Honey,"John said, as he helped her lie down. "Everything is going to be just fine. You'll see."

"It's going to be just fine for you," she snapped. "But I'm not so sure about me." Another groan from Eileen made John jump. He stood anxiously by her side.

"I'm going to go and see if we can get you something for that pain." I said, looking into John's worried face. "In the meantime what I'd like you to do, if you can, is help your wife with those relaxation exercises that you practiced in the pre-natal classes."

He gave Eileen one of the stuffed toys to hold as he nodded to me. "We'll give it our best shot." He planted a kiss on his Eileen's forehead, "Won't we love?"

I hurried along the corridor to the desk to report to the charge nurse. Mrs.Hummel listened to my brief report before going down to check on my patient's progress. As a student nurse, I was only allowed to do the initial admission of the patients and assist the registered staff where I was needed.

The charge nurse returned to the desk. "You can go and do the admission now. I've given Mrs.Gibbs something for her pain."

When I went back to Eileen's room, I found John busily unpacking his wife's suitcase. I looked at him and shook my head. "There's no need to do all that; this isn't the room that your wife will be coming back to once she's had her baby."

"Well," John snapped,"I've got to do something. My wife has told me she can manage this birthing thing on her own. And here I was thinking that I was going to be able to help."

Looking into his strong, oval shaped, angry face, I felt sorry for him. Eileen gasped, and muttered. "Oh! This really hurts."

"How are you doing there?" I gently touched her round glistened cheek.

"It's certainly a lot different than when we practiced." Her brown eyes looked up at me. "Do you have any children?"

John came and stood beside me. "What difference does it make if she has?"

"It makes all the difference in the world," Eileen yelled. "She would know what I'm going through right now, and would understand, while you never can."

"Okay! Okay folks." I looked at both of them. "This isn't going to be easy for either one of you, but believe me you are both going to get through it."

John had taken a cloth and gently wiped his wife's perspiring face. "I'm so sorry Love. I hate to see you hurting so much."

Eileen looked sleepily into her husband's eyes. The pain medication had begun to take effect. She grasped his hands. "I'm sorry too." She mumbled. "And I don't think you're useless."

"Well!" I said."I have all I need for now so I will leave you both alone for a little while. If you need anything just use the Call-Bell and I will be right in."

Several hours passed before Eileen was ready to have her baby. With the help of an epidural and some more medication, she had been able to rest. John had benefited from a little sleep as well.

Now everything was on the move again. As we wheeled Eileen into the delivery room, she let out a loud shriek. John wrung his hands, and looked dismayed as he blurted out. "What have I done? It wasn't supposed to be like this."

One of the other staff members quickly took him in hand. She propelled John down to the father's waiting area to get changed and prepped.

In the delivery room things moved swiftly. Eileen was placed on the special bed and her feet placed into stirrups; her perineum was cleansed and then draped with sterile cloths. While this was being done, the attending obstetrician came into the room.

After inspecting his patient's progress he said, "You can go and bring in Mr. Gibbs."

John was all ready, fully dressed in his scrubbed greens with his head covered. I beckoned to him to come with me.

"Now, just remember," I said, putting a finger to my lips. "You must keep absolutely quiet while you're in there. Your wife's obstetrician does not tolerate anyone making a noise. Do you understand, John?"

"Of course I do." He nodded. "You won't hear a peep out of me."

Taking him gently by the arm, I guided him into the delivery room. At a quick glance I saw that the baby's head was visible and that the birth was near.

John stopped dead, as we entered the room. His eyes above his mask opened wide, and he gasped loudly. I still had a firm grip of his arm, which was a good thing, because John turned towards the doctor and yelled. " Don't you dare look at my wife when she's all uncovered like that."

For a brief moment there was an uncanny hush, then the attending obstetrician angrily shouted. "Get that man out of here. Get him out of my sight, right now....

When she heard this Eileen started to weep loudly. Some of us present tried to get the doctor to change his mind but he flatly refused to listen to any of our pleas.

John did not leave willingly. "Look, I'm sorry, really sorry. Please, please, just let me stay," he said, as I moved him towards the door.

I sat with him until after his baby was delivered. He was beyond consoling so we sat there not saying anything. I thought that the only reason he had behaved that way was he'd been overwhelmed by all that was taking place.

Still, I felt compelled to ask him why he would act in the manner he had. "What on earth did you think you were doing when you yelled like that at your wife's doctor?"

His dark eyes glinted. "I didn't like the way he was looking at her body."

"What! My loud exclamation made him wince.

"It wasn't right that he was staring at her like that."

I grinned. "Oh! John." I gently patted his arm. "John, how on earth do you think he was going to deliver your baby? He had to look at her to make sure that she and your child were okay."

With his head hanging down, he mumbled, "I know that. I know."

Eileen delivered a healthy 7lb 2oz baby boy, and while she was waiting to be taken to her postpartum room John was allowed to see them both. His disappointment over not seeing the birth was soon forgotten as he reveled in being a proud father and an attentive husband. He gently touched his son's tiny hands and lovingly kissed his wife.

I have often wondered whether John ever recalls what he did in the delivery room that day. I believe that if he ever needs one his son's birthday should act as a reminder of this extraordinary event.

When You've Got an Itch

I was alone in the hallway of the chronic care facility when I suddenly heard a female voice. "Help me. Please, someone help me."

It was not easy to pinpoint where this call was coming from, as there were many rooms on this ward. The voice again called out. "Please...please...isn't they're anyone out there."

It was obvious this person was in distress but who and where was she. Why hadn't she used the call bell system?

After looking in several rooms, I came to Ruth's door. "This is just terrible, " the woman's voice cried from the room. "Where is everybody?"

I pushed open the door and found a female propped up in a specially designed wheelchair. Her hands lay awkwardly in front of her. She was trying to get her mouth around a calling tube but it had slipped to the side and out of her reach.

"Oh! Thank goodness, "Ruth exclaimed, " I was beginning to think everyone had been carried away by Aliens, or something, and I was here alone!"

I smiled at this lady's sense of humor. Her dark oval features frowned as she looked at me.

"Umm...."She said, "Haven't seen you before. Are you new here?"

Nodding, I said, "Yes, I've only been here a couple of weeks."

After I had given her my name, she inquired, "So what are you?"

"You mean professionally?" I said.

"Yes!" Ruth said with a deep sigh.

"Is it important to you?" I asked.

She sighed again. "I used to be a nurse once myself. Now look at me."

Then you will understand why I need to find out why you were calling out. You sounded desperate.""

Ruth gave a little giggle, and she grinned. "Would you believe that I've gone and forgotten what I wanted?"

She chuckled. "You must be thinking who is this odd person?"

I smiled at her. "No, I don't think that you're odd at all."

"Well there is something you can do for me now that I've got you here, "she said. "Please would you put my call device closer to my mouth so I can get a hold of it.'

While I adjusted the device for her I asked, "So, how long have you been in this institution?"

"Too long, " she quickly replied.

Ruth looked into my face that was now close to her own. Her brown eyes closely scrutinizing me. "You've got a nice complexion. That must be all that good English blood you've got, just like me." She winked saucily at me.

I laughed, and shook my head. "I'm not sure you're right in your assumption about us having any special kind of blood, but hey, you never know, you could be right."

Ruth laughed. "Well, we at least have the same roots."

She looked quizzical as she continued. "You haven't answered my earlier question. What level of nurse are you?"

"I am a nurse's aide now, but I hope some day to take a course and become a registered caregiver, " I told her.

"Well, as I was saying earlier I used to be a Registered Nurse. I took my training in England and worked there as well as here in Canada. I loved being a nurse." Her voice trembled.

Ruth moved her head as if trying to point to a cupboard door. "My old nurse's uniform is hanging up in that cupboard."

Opening the door, I saw her navy blue, red-lined cloak on one hanger. Underneath it was her nurse's dress and apron. Her hat was in a plastic bag on the shelf.

Ruth was quiet while I was looking at these things. Then speaking in a soft voice she said, " I could have still been a nurse if I'd been a bit more careful."

I looked with curiosity at her. "What do you mean if you'd been more careful? What did you do?"

Before she had a chance to answer Ruth's face grimaced and she started to violently twitch her nose. "Now I remember what it was that I wanted, " she said, trying to shake her head. "My nose is driving me nuts today. It's so itchy, and there's no way I can scratch it myself; will you please do it for me?"

Obliging this cheerful middle-aged woman, I gently rubbed the top of her nose and around the sides of her face. She sighed. "Oh! That feels so much better already. Thanks!"

"It's murder when that happens, " Ruth added. "Luckily it does not do it very often or I would really go crazy. It's such a stupid little thing, and yet it's something I can't even do."

I sensed from her voice the feeling of frustration she was experiencing at not being able to perform this small task herself. I gently touched her limp hands. "Well, I can't imagine what it must be like not being able to use your own hands. It must be a very hard handicap to live with?"

Ruth looked wistfully at me. She nodded. "You're right it is hard sometimes living like this. When I was a nurse I helped many patients in similar situations. I never thought I'd be in the same position one day myself."'

"What happened to you?" I asked.

Ruth shook her head. "I'd really rather not talk about it, if you don't mind?"

"That's okay with me." I told her. "But if you ever do want to borrow an ear to blow off steam, and I'm on duty, please feel free to call me."

She smiled. "I'll remember that."

"I'll report the problem you're having today, with that itch, to the head-nurse. We should be able to get something to put on it that will ease the irritation."

"That sounds like a good idea." Ruth bent over towards her mouth device. "And, that's better, now I can reach it."

14

"When I've got time maybe we can chat a bit more?" I walked towards to the door and waved as I left.

As I made my way down to the nurse's station I felt sadness that this simple act of being able to scratch, that all of us take for granted was now denied this lady. I also hoped that something would be prescribed to give her the relief she deserved.

Just knowing wasn't Enough

Mrs. Green's oval features were lit up with a broad grin. She approached the desk prepared to be admitted.

"Well, " she said, "as you can all see, here I am again back for another visit." She placed her documents on the counter.

"You must get tired of having me in here so often?" I smiled and shook my head. "No that's not true. In fact you are a great help to us."

Mrs. Green over the past year had been a patient many times on our medical unit. The staff had got to know a lot about her and her family. She also knew most of us by our first names as well as some of our personal history.

"Who'll be admitting me today?" Mrs. Green cheerily asked. She laughed." I could probably fill out my own forms. I've been here so much"

I owned up that I would be the one doing her paperwork. "That's fine, " she told me. "Just give me a few minutes before you come down to see me. I'd like to get myself settled in first."

"No problem, " I said.

Mrs. Green was a charming woman in her early fifties. She'd been widowed for several years and had no children. Her primary cancer nearly twenty years earlier had been in her breast but now it was in her right lung. It was to have some treatments arranged for this that she was back on the ward.

When I walked into her room, I found her sitting and gazing out of the window.

"Hello Mrs. Green. What do you think of the view from this room? You can see a lot of the city from here."

"It's very nice." She gave a deep sigh. " But oh! I do wish that these new treatments were all over and done with."

"You sound tired, " I said." How do you feel?"

"To be honest nurse...., I'm not really sure, " she replied.

Looking closely at her, I saw what I had missed before at the desk. The dark circles under her brown eyes; the wan drawn appearance of her face. She looked exhausted.

"Would you like to have a rest before we begin?" I asked. "I can get a lot of the information from your old charts. Then I'll come back later to fill in the rest"

She nodded. " I don't know why I'm so tired. But, if it's not going to upset your routine too much I'd like to do that. A nap should set things right."

This was the first time I had ever seen her looking so weary. I hoped that it wasn't due to some other underlying problem she might have.

Mrs. Green was one of those warm, friendly persons who had the marvelous ability to relate to all sorts of people. It was a pleasure to know her, and care for her.

Her special gift though was relating well with other cancer patients. Whenever she was on the ward we could always rely on her to talk to any patient suffering from the same condition as her.

Nurses learn a lot of theory in school about cancer but sometimes knowing about it is not enough. That is why people as Mrs. Green were a Godsend to us. Their own personal experiences were so helpful, especially to patients newly diagnosed. They seem to cope better if they could talk to someone facing the same problem they were.

Nonetheless, I was concerned why Mrs. Green's health had deteriorated so much. I wondered what was happening with her to cause this amount of change. She had gone through so much already, and didn't need anything else to go wrong.

Returning later to see her, I found her up. She was busy eating her supper. She smiled, as I bent towards her meal tray to check its contents.

"I wouldn't get that close to it, " she said with a little laugh, " it's lasagna and it's got a lot of garlic in it. It's good, but I'll have to keep from breathing on anyone for awhile."

17

I laughed with her. It pleased me to see that she was more her usual jovial self.

After completing her admission paper work, I was about to leave her room when she said, "Nurse, even though I'm not feeling as perky as I'd like to be. Please let me still talk with any patients who could use my help?"

"That's very generous of you Mrs. Green, " I smiled. "And I'll remember that."

Her pale features glowed as she told me, "I really don't mind doing it. In fact I enjoy it."

Mrs. Green grinned. "I know all you nurses are kind and caring but you can't always give a patient what they need. It's much easier talking with someone who has the same disease and knows how they're feeling."

"I'm sure it is, " I said. "And, as I've told you Mrs. Green, many times, your help is very much appreciated."

During that particular period, this dear lady visited with two newly diagnosed patients, and several others in for chemotherapy treatment. Even though her own health wasn't the best she was always upbeat and smiling. It was as if by helping others she had found an inner strength and a purpose. It was a good thing for her to do. It was also good for us to see because it reminded us we were not the only ones with caring skills.

Finding the Courage

"Don't you dare put on that big light, " he snarled. "I can see all I want to see of myself with just the small one on."

David Barn was in his late thirties and he was a farmer. I'd learned from his chart that he wasn't coping well with his accident.

As I drew closer to him, I was able to see that he was sitting propped up in his bed. Bending my head slightly towards him, I tried to make eye contact.

"I understand." I said. "Why you might not like the room lit up but I need to be able to see you if I'm going to provide you with any care today."

"I don't want anyone touching me, " he growled. "So that means that you can just go away and leave me alone."

"Mr. Barn, " I said, "or do you prefer to be called David?" As he didn't answer I continued. "You know that you have to have certain things done for you, so I can't leave."

He pulled the covers up tightly around his neck. Glaring at me, he yelled. "You people just don't get it do you. I want to be left alone. I'm no good to anyone anymore."

"I don't believe that for one minute, "I said. "As I am your nurse today I have to follow your doctor's instructions or both of us will be in deep trouble. You because your legs won't heal as they should and me because I failed to obey orders.

David made no comment to what I had said.

I was ahead with my other work, so I pulled up a chair beside his bed and sat down. "I'm sorry that you feel so bad about what's happened to you, but if your legs are ever going to heal properly so you can..."

"So I can what?" he shouted.

"So you can get those two prosthetic legs fitted, " I quietly answered.

"So you can get those two prosthetic legs fitted, " he said sarcastically, mimicking me.

"Look David, " I said, "you're angry right now, but I have a job to do and one way or another it's going to get done. We are all here to help you. I believe you know that."

"How would you feel, " David muttered, " if you had both your legs hacked off, and you couldn't get around anymore. You suddenly became half a person?"

"I'm not sure how I'd feel. But, I do know I'd try very hard to look at what I still had and not just at what I'd lost."

He peered crossly at me. "Yeah! Yeah! That sounds all so high and mighty, but you can still stand up. I can't." David's voice broke. He took in a big gulp of air as he tried to catch his breath, and recover his composure.

"Perhaps, " I said, "if I told you that you're not the first person I've met who had both legs amputated, and had to learn to walk all over again when he got his new legs, how would you feel then?"

"I would say you were just making it all up, " he snapped.

"No David, " I said, shaking my head. "I'm not making it up. I'm talking about the World War 11 fighter pilot, Douglas Bader. He visited the hospital in England where I was working and I got to meet him. He lost both his legs in a flying accident. He didn't let that stop him from living a full life."

"Well, I'm not him. I don't fly planes. I have a farm to run."

"I know that. What I am trying to tell you is that you have a choice. You can either let this accident ruin your whole life or you can look at it as another challenge to overcome as Bader did."

"I'd like to be able to do that, but at the moment I can't. Do you understand?"

"Yes David, " I said. "Just give yourself a little more time, it will get easier. If you like I can get a social worker to come in and talk things over with you."

20

"No. No, that's not necessary, " David said. "But thank-you anyway for the offer."

I stood up and placed a hand on his arm. "I want to help you David, but you need to let me get on with my work."

"Well, " he muttered, " do what you have to. I still don't want to see them."

It was not easy providing this patient with care in a dimly lit room, but I respected his wishes. I knew that re-wrapping his stumps was going to be difficult unless I could see well. It was also important to examine his incisions to assess how they were healing.

"David, I will have to put on the other light, "I gently told him. But you don't have to look at what I'm doing unless you want to."

"I've already told you I don't want to have to look at them."

"That's okay, "I said. You lay back down and I'll just do what I have to."

It took nearly a week of gentle coaxing from his caregivers and his family before David would agree to look at his lower limbs. When he finally did he was surprised to see that they were not as ugly, or as short as he'd feared.

"That harvester did a real number on me, " he said, " but I guess it could have been worse. I could have died."

I smiled. "I'm glad you didn't, " I told him. "I wouldn't have met you."

David smiled broadly. "Yeah! But, they, " he touched the end of his right stump. "They do not look half as bad as I imagined they would.

When the man from the prosthetic department came in to see him, David was in a jovial mood. It was good to see this positive change in him. He jokingly said to us, "Maybe I'll go for something that makes me a bit taller."

It was suggested, however, that this wasn't such a good idea as it could affect his balance. David was able to accept what he was told. He just shrugged his shoulders and raised his eyebrows as he murmured, " that's okay. I wouldn't want to be seen staggering all over the place that's for sure."

He jokingly added, " just don't make me any shorter than I was that's all. I wouldn't want my wife towering over me."

Before David was fitted with his prosthesis, I was assigned to a different clinical area. However, I went back several weeks later to inquire after him. I was informed that after several small setbacks David Barn had been discharged home.

In all my years of nursing practice, I never saw anyone accept the loss of a body part easily. David had found it that much more difficult, because of his fears that he would not be able to provide anymore for his family.

I was glad to hear from the head-nurse, that before he was discharged David had accepted the truth about himself. He'd learned that he wasn't any less a man because of his accident, and that his disability didn't have to limit him with what he could still do.

A Sharing of Pain

The emergency ward of any hospital is a very busy area. Working in the ER can be exciting, but sometimes it is mentally exhausting as well as physically draining.

Peter was brought in after having been run over by a truck. He was riding his motor bike and had crossed over an intersection when the accident occurred. He was seriously injured and in a lot of pain.

While the doctors were trying to save his life, I was given the task to comfort his mother. She was very distraught. Since I also had a son of my own who as hers rode a motor bike, this allowed me to relate to her intense emotional distress. I knew how I would feel had the same thing happened to my son.

We were sitting in the special room allotted for trauma family members. "I don't know what I'm going to do, " she sobbed. "Lord, please don't let him die. He's all I've got in this world."

"What about your husband?" I gently asked.

"What about him?" she cried aloud. " He isn't here is here? Do you see him anyplace?"

It was obvious by the tone of her voice that this was another underlying problem. I chose not to give her an answer.

Peter's mother started to move towards the door. "I want to see my son, " she said. "What's taking them so long?"

I gently took her arm." The doctors are busy with him right now, " I said helping her back to her seat. "Once they have him comfortable, I know they will come and get you."

"I told him not to ride that bike in the dark, " she sobbed, " but he wouldn't listen to me. Why is it our children never listen to us? Have you any children?" she asked me.

"Yes, " I told her." I have a daughter and a son."

"Do they listen to you? Do they do as you tell them to?" She looked into my face.

I shook my head. "No, they don't always listen to what I say. But then do any children?"

"Well what if your son wanted to ride his bike in the dark. Would you let him? Would you try to stop him?" Peter's mother's tear-stained face glared at me.

I swallowed hard before speaking. "It just so happens that my son does ride a motor-bike and I................."

"You wouldn't let him go out at night, would you?" she quickly interrupted.

"I should have stopped him, " she cried. "I know one thing for sure, once he's recovered he'll never ride that dammed bike ever again."

Just then, the supervisor came into the room. She motioned to me with a slight movement of her head; then she came over to Peter's mother and sat down beside her.

"Mrs. Starr, " she said gently. "You can come and see your son now. But first I need to tell you something about his condition. He's been severely injured as you know and he's in......."

Peter's mother was on her feet and heading out of the door. "I want to see my son, " she yelled. " I don't care what any of you say. He's going to be all right. I just know that he's going to be fine."

I followed Peter's mother as she headed towards the room that held her son. The supervisor informed me that Peter wasn't expected to live. I would have to give Mrs. Starr all the support she was going to need as well as call the Special Services for some additional help.

The hospital had an excellent Pastoral Service department and I was able to relay to them that they would soon be required in the ER department.

When the supervisor and I entered Peter's room we found his mother loudly sobbing with her arms splayed across her son's body. I moved over to her and gently placed my own arm around her.

24

"He can't die, " she wailed. "He's too young. He hasn't had enough time to live."

"I'm so sorry, " I said, my own eyes now filling with tears. I wasn't sure what I should do. As a nursing student, I had been told it was best not to get too emotionally involved in patient's problems, which was what I was doing.

I looked at the supervisor and she shook her head. She then whispered something to me that I've never forgotten. "It's alright to let Peter's mother see that you share her pain, and your tears shows her that you really care."

And share it we did over the course of the next hour holding onto each other, praying and crying together. Mrs. Starr later came back to the hospital to see me after her son's funeral and she thanked me for my support. Although this occurred while I was in the role of a nurse it was more an act of one mother empathizing with another's suffering.

Minus Some Toes

"Oh! My goodness, " I loudly exclaimed, "I don't believe this. How on earth could this have happened?"

I shook my head with disbelief as I stared at the sight that I had uncovered. "I've never in my life ever seen anything like it."

"What's the matter with you?" Mrs. Bell snapped crossly. "What are you staring at down there?"

Mrs. Bell was usually a cheerful, pleasant lady, so her outburst surprised me. I had looked after her many times in the Chronic Care Institution and was familiar with her numerous health problems. Nevertheless, nothing had prepared me for this.

I quickly placed the covers back over my patient's legs and feet. "It's nothing really, " I said. I tried to sound calm as I asked, "How do you feel today?"

"Why are you asking me that, " she snapped. "You know I've got lots of things wrong with me and I seldom get a day I can enjoy anymore, " she said with a sob.

"Oh! Mrs. Bell, " I gently patted her hand, "I know it can't be easy for you with all your health problems, and I'm really sorry if I've upset you."

I tried to give her hand a gentle squeeze, but she pulled it out of the way.

She sniffed. "I don't think I'll bother getting up this morning, if that's fine with you? I don't know what it is today, but somehow I do feel different."

"I nodded and smiled. "That's perfectly okay with me, you probably should stay in bed all day today."

She gave me an odd look. "Now why would I want to do that? I've never done that before."

"Let's leave it for now, Mrs. Bell, " I said. "I have to go and get the Registered Nurse first, to check something out for me."

She stared at me inquiringly. "If you don't mind?" I said.

"Why do you have to do that?" she said hotly. "All the staff here are well aware of all the things I have wrong with me."

I shook my head "Yes, they probably do. But, something weird has happened to your left foot and it has to be reported right away."

"What's happened to it?" She glared at me.

I took a big gulp before answering. I wasn't sure if I should be telling this lady what had happened to her foot. "Em....em.....em.." I muttered.

"Oh! For the love of goodness, " Mrs. Bell sat up straight in her bed and started to pull at the covers. "What is the big deal? I already know I've got some purple toes."

"No don't do that" I said, as I quickly stopped her from disturbing the blankets.

"Well, " she sat with her arms crossed, "If I can't see for myself what's wrong then you've got to tell me."

Looking into my elderly patient's flushed angry looking features I knew I had to tell her something.

Mrs. Bell, " I said, "You know how you've had that bad circulation problem, in your feet for awhile now. Well, last night sometime......."

"Last night sometime, what?" she interrupted. I know that there's been something wrong with them for a long time. Now tell me what I don't know."

"You know how your toes on that foot had all turned black, " I said, "and they were giving you a lot of pain"

"Yes, yes, yes I know all that, " she snapped, "And, it was damned painful."

"Well how does your foot feel now?" I watched her closely to assess her response.

She sat quietly for a minute and then giving a giggle said, " Now that you've asked me, it's funny but it feels better today. Why is that?"

I swallowed hard, then said. "Your toes are in your bed Mrs. Bell."

"Of course they are, " she laughed, "and so are both my feet."

It was at that moment that the Registered Nurse popped her head around the door. "How is everything going in here?" she asked.

"Oh! " I said with relief, "Am I ever pleased to see you. I was just coming to get you. There's something here I have to show you."

Mrs. Bell smiled. "Yes, seems there's something wrong with my toes." She chortled. "As If you didn't know that."

Looking back at this incident it still leaves me amazed at what the body is capable of doing. This dear lady's gangrenous toes had all fallen off sometime during the night, and she seemed to be unaffected by it.

When Mrs. Bell was told the news she was understandably shocked, so was the RN when she removed the bedclothes?

"Oh! My goodness, " she loudly exclaimed.

"Let me see them, I want to look, " Mrs. Bell demanded. To appease her the RN allowed her to see her foot.

Strangely enough, after that, this patient's left foot looked much improved. It healed up nicely, which was remarkable, considering her circulatory status and that she was in her late seventies.

Later, Mrs. Bell, got a lot of pleasure telling patients what had happened to her, and watching for the shocked responses. Because, as she would always add, "You know what happened to me was quite unique." She had that right. In addition, thankfully, I never saw it ever repeated in all my years of nursing.

A Valuable Lesson

"I hate you, "the young boy screamed, as he tried to wriggle free from my firm grasp. As I'd been instructed by the head nurse to take him to the special area for changing burn dressings I wasn't about to let him get free. I knew if that happened I'd be in deep trouble.

Yet there was a part of me that did not want to put this small person through the ordeal that I knew was coming. Nevertheless, it had to be done or his burns would never heal. I began to wonder how I was ever going to manage this task I'd been assigned.

"I hate you, " he spat the words out again.

"Please Bobby, "I said, " you know that you have to have your dressings changed. You've been having them done often enough so why are you acting up like this now?"

Bobby had been playing in the kitchen in his home and he had knocked a pot of boiling water over himself. He had several nasty, third-degree burns around his left arm and upper torso. With the care he'd been getting and his own natural affinity for fast healing they were coming along nicely.

The small features scrunched up as he began to sob. "They're going to hurt me. I don't want to be hurt. Let go of me. I want my mum. I want my mother." He yelled this out so loud that a few other children on the ward stopped what they were doing and moved towards us.

Oh! Lord, I thought, please help me here. This is way too difficult for me to manage on my own.

As if by a miracle, another nurse suddenly appeared beside us. Susan was one of the regular staff members on the pediatric unit and was used to dealing with these kinds of problems. I was very happy to see her.

"What's all this racket about?" Susan muttered crossly She arched her brows at me as she looked for a response.

"Bobby doesn't want to go and have his dressings done, " I said, " and I'm not sure I feel good about trying to drag him down to that room."

"Oh! Is that so." She said scornfully. "Well when you work on this unit you'll find that you often have to do things as that. You need to remember that with children we often have to be what may seem cruel in order to be kind. If we didn't they would never get better.

Susan lightly brushed at the tears on Bobby's face. "It's not always easy, " she said, " but that's just the way it is. So you might as well get used to hearing kids making a fuss and crying."

Bobby was now yelling and screaming at the top of his lungs. We also had several other children standing around us who had come to see what was going on.

"That's it, " Susan loudly grumbled, "you're making far too much fuss Bobby. You are not helping yourself or the others with this racket. So enough, already." Susan peered into the small tear stained face then gently patted him on the head.

She scowled at the group of small, interested onlookers. "The rest of you kids get back in your rooms while I take care of this young man." Taking a firm grip of him, she propelled him down the hall.

I tried to get the other children into their respective rooms, but even that was a difficult task, as I hadn't a clue of any of their names or their rooms. Eventually by checking name tags and with giggling help from them I did manage to get them all back safely.

When Susan came marching back to the desk, I was preparing some of the gruel that several of the infants were supposed to eat. "Well, " she said sarcastically, " you should be able to at least do that without my having to bail you out."

I chose not to make any comment and continued with what I was doing. This was my first experience on a pediatric unit and at that moment I was thinking it would also be my last.

30

I heard Bobby coming back up the hall. He was still crying and as he passed the desk I took a quick peek at his face. He looked to me like the unhappiest little person I'd ever seen. My instinct was to go and try and comfort him but as Susan was the one pushing his wheelchair I sat still.

Later together, with not too much trouble, we got all the children fed. Just when I had started to think that I might like working again on this ward, as most of the children were really cute, I had that notion flattened.

I'd been told to go and settle the children in the room that housed those who had the croup. There were five cots each encased in a huge plastic tent. Inside each one sat a small, sobbing, sorrowful looking child.

All of their parents had recently left so I assumed that much of their distress was due to them now being on their own. I popped my upper body in under the first steamy, hot covering and started to try and pacify its occupant.

The crying did begin to ease as I gently sponged the small girl and made her comfortable. While I was busy doing this the other four children had continued to serenade us with their loud cries.

As I moved over to the next cot I thought, well that's one down and only four more to go. But as soon as I'd left the first child she immediately joined in the chorus with her roommates. The noise that those tiny people made was one tremendous racket.

Again, Susan appeared on the scene. She quickly scanned the room and giving me a look of disgust, she let out a yell that was so loud it must have been heard on all the other floors in the hospital.

However, after that every one of the small figures who had been screaming and crying sat silently in their cots. It was truly amazing to see this but it wasn't something that I could do.

Susan peered into my face. "That's the only way to do it to get them all quiet." She then added, "Going from one to one trying to pacify each of them individually is no good. It just doesn't work."

"Now you should be able to at least get them settled, " she muttered crossly, before flouncing out of the room.

Since this experience, I recognize that the nurses who have chosen pediatrics as their area of expertise are unique. Nevertheless, with what I had seen and faced I had no doubts that I would never be any good working on that unit. I would not be coming back. It was however for me a good learning experience.

For Whom did the Bell Toll?

I was most fortunate in my years of nursing to have had a wide and varied level of experiences. During the time when I was back at nursing school I also worked as a casual help in an active treatment hospital. This kind of staff member gets to work in many different areas of a hospital. Such work can be very taxing on a person because one never knows what the atmosphere of any given ward will be like. Often one would be given the worst assignments and/or the head-nurse might have certain rare peculiarities. This is a story of such a person and her bell.

When I checked in with the nursing office that day I learned that I was to go to the orthopedic floor. The patients on that ward were usually heavy, meaning they required a lot of care, or they'd be having hip or knee replacements. As I made my way up to the floor to report for duty I was preparing myself for a very busy shift.

Arriving on the ward, I quickly scanned the rooms trying to assess the patient load. All the beds appeared to be filled but there were several patients walking in the halls so at that moment it didn't look as bad as I'd feared.

There were several staff members at the nurse's station. As I greeted them I said, " I'm your casual help today."

"Well were certainly glad to see you, " an older looking nurse said to me. I'm Susan and this is Pat and this is Dorothy." She pointed to the others.

After telling them my name I volunteered that I had worked on that kind of ward before.

Just then, a tall business-like woman appeared at the desk. I was informed that she was the head-nurse. She gave me a brief glance as she picked up several sheets of paper and moved

33

away from that area. Susan beckoned to me that we were all supposed to follow her.

We made our way down the hall and into a small lounge. I figured that this must be where we would be having the report and receive our assignments.

After each shift, each nurse gives a report of the status of the patients assigned to him/her for period. This report could be given either on tape or by verbal communication. Thankfully I saw that we would be listening to a taped report that day.

The head-nurse positioned herself at the top of the table and motioned to the rest of us to sit down. Looking at her nametag pinned to her pristine starched uniform I saw she was called Mrs. F. Baker.

Mrs. Baker scanned each patient's name in the patient's card index and quickly assigned him or her to the different nurses. She looked up at me. I've been told you've worked on an orthopedic unit before, so you know what to expect. Is that correct?"

I nodded, "Yes I have but......"

"I do not want to hear any buts Mrs., " she glanced over at my name tag, "Stirling is it."

"Yes that's right but I was just going to say....."

"Do you have a problem with hearing?"

I shook my head as Mrs.Baker added, "I'm pleased to hear that perhaps now we can get on with the report. These will be your patients for today." She pushed a sheet of paper towards me with six names listed on it.

"If you need to know anymore about them, " Mrs. Baker said, " then you can check with the staff nurse after you've heard the report. Now if there're no more interruptions let us hear what the night staff have to say."

As I made my way down the hall towards my patient's rooms, Susan touched me on the arm. "Don't let Mrs.Baker's attitude get to you. She's really not as bad as she may seem."

"Well, " I turned towards her, "I think I'll wait and see how the day turns out. Anyway, it looks as if I am going to be very busy so the time should pass quickly. See you later perhaps."

Susan carried on down the hall while I walked into the first room listed on my sheet.

Mrs. Green was going to have a hip replacement so I needed to finish her prep. She was an elderly lady and she was obviously afraid.

"Oh! Am I glad to see you nurse. I don't think I can go for my surgery today. I just don't feel well."

"What is the matter?" I stood by her bed looking down at her, noting that her color did look a little grey but that she seemed to be breathing fine.

"I don't know, " her voice wavered as she spoke, " I don't want to go for this operation. Maybe I won't wake up once they put me to sleep." A tear trickled down her full, rounded face.

"Mrs. Green, " I placed my hand in hers. "It's normal to feel the way you do but there's really no other recourse for you." As I was talking to her she began to squeeze my fingers.

"Whoa!" I pulled my hand free from hers. "You certainly have nothing wrong with your hands. That's quite the grip you have."

Somewhere in the distance, I heard a bell being rung incessantly. It didn't sound to me as a patient's call bell, but as I wasn't a regular member of the floor staff I thought I'd better go and see if it came from any of my assigned rooms.

"Mrs.Green, " I said. "I have to go and see where that noise is coming from. I promise I'll be back soon."

As I came out of this patient's room the sound grew even louder. What on earth was that?

I looked at the outside lights of my other rooms and saw no signs that it was coming from any of them. This was very odd.

Susan appeared and pointed down the hall. "You're supposed to go to the desk."

"Me, " I asked her. "What for? And what on earth is that racket. It's like no other bell I've ever heard."

Susan smiled and nodded, "You're right about that, but yes it's ringing for you."

"I haven't got the time right now to go running to the desk. I've got a lot of work to do and I've just got started."

"Look, " Susan pointed towards the nurse's station, " Mrs. Baker is waiting for you to go to see her.

"Am I hearing you correctly? I'm supposed to drop everything and run down to the desk whenever that bell sounds?" My surprised tone again evoked a smile from Susan.

"Yup! That's the way we work on this floor. We all have a special signal and that's yours."

"Well how the heck is a newcomer supposed to know that." I said crossly. The sound of the bell seemed to be getting louder.

"You'd better go and see what she wants." Susan gently pushed me in the direction of the desk. "I'll keep an eye on your patients till you get back."

Mrs. Baker scowled at me as I approached the desk. By now she had stopped the ringing. As she laid the bell on the counter I could see that it was a medium sized hand-bell.

"You obviously do have a hearing problem after all Mrs. Stirling, " Her sarcastic tone irked me even more than knowing I was not doing my job.

"What makes you say that?" I retorted back.

"Because you didn't come immediately when I rang for you. You are expected to come as soon as you hear my signal."

"What was it you wanted?" I looked her straight in the eyes.

"Nothing in particular only to see if you would come when I called. That's all!"

I took a deep breath and as I have rarely been intimidated, I let this head-nurse know how I felt.

"I am here to work Mrs. Baker, not to be answering a silly bell. And just for the record I was never informed that this was a common practice on this floor."

It was obvious that this head-nurse rarely, if ever, had anyone question what she did. She glowered at me. "Your attitude leaves much to be desired, and I will be reporting all of this to the Director of Nursing."

Looking her squarely in the face I said, "That's just fine with me. Now if there's nothing more..." Mrs. Baker shook her head.

36

"Then, " I said, " I'll be getting back to my work. I've got a ton of things to do."

Several off the regular staff had been watching this heated exchange. As I made my way back down the hall Pat and Dorothy gave me a thumbs up sign.

During that shift, the ringing sound was heard often, but I simply ignored it. I never did go back to work on that floor nor did I have to report to the Director. This made me wonder if my outburst had had some effect and perhaps someone else had spoken up about that bell. Anyway, I would like to think that's what happened.

Privacy Is Always Important

I glowered at the orderly. What he was doing to the elderly male patient was contrary to everything I'd been taught.

During the Registered Nursing Assistant's program, part of the practical work application was in a veteran's hospital. The long wards reminded me very much of the hospital layouts in England. Metal beds were lined up in regimental fashion down each side of the unit.

The patients who lived in this institution had all served at some time in the armed forces. Because they had all been in the military, where living conditions were often overcrowded, some of the orderlies wrongly assumed that these men lacked any pride or self-respect.

Mr. Kent was part of my assignment, and when he found out that I had served for a short time in the Women's Royal Navy, he would tease me by saying, "You know, you're an old veteran like me." Yet, compared to the many years he had served, my service time was minor.

The ward had no separate cubicles, or curtains between the beds. It was, however, important to us students that when we provided our patients with care that their privacy be respected. Mr. Kent loved to josh me on this issue as well. "It's real nice nurse, the way you make sure I'm all covered up before giving me my bed-bath. The orderlies here don't ever do that."

"Well, " I said. "It's the way we have been taught and it's the way it's supposed to be done. It only takes a fraction more time, and it's also much nicer for you."

His round weathered face beamed. "It's fine with me nurse. I just don't want you going to too much trouble on my account." I smiled. "It's no trouble at all."

Chuckling he gave me a cheeky grin. "You've really got me all covered up this time, so how are you going to give me a bath?"

I shook my head. "It'll be as easy as falling off a log. You just wait and see."

Mr. Kent called across to his buddy in the next bed. "How about this, Charlie, I'm getting the royal treatment this morning. What do you think of that?"

The man in the next bed was being bathed by one of the orderlies, and he had him completely uncovered. Charlie lay on top of his bed nude and fully exposed. "Okay. " Charlie called back, " I'm sure that we haven't got anything that your nurse hasn't seen before, so what's all her fussing about."

That way of thinking bothered me, because even though nurses do get to look at many fully unclothed bodies of both sexes, it still doesn't mean they want to see someone's bare body when it's unnecessary. I turned away from the sight of the naked man in the next bed and carried on with Mr. Kent's care.

"Nurse." My patient said. " Even though I've been teasing you about being fussy when you're doing my bath, I want you to know, it is really enjoyable."

He beamed. "I haven't felt so warm and cozy while getting washed in years. You're doing a tip-top job. He gave a contented sigh and snuggled further down under the warm, flannel blanket.

The following day when I walked into this ward I found Mr. Kent's bed empty. I was worried that something unforeseen had happened to him. After making some inquiries about his whereabouts, I was told, "it was Mr. Kent's special bath day, and that the orderly had taken him down to the tub room."

This man was my only patient, so I felt I had a right to go and see how he was doing. Not being shy about approaching this room, I knocked on the tub-room door and went in. The sight that met my eyes made me furious. I glowered at the orderly, and I stared in disbelief at what was happening.

Mr. Kent was lying on a stone slab, not a stitch of clothing on his person and he was being hosed down.

Trying to quell my temper, I angrily muttered. "What! What do you think you are doing here?"

"What does it look like I'm doing? "the orderly snarled sarcastically.

I bristled at his tone and his lack of any interest for my patient's dignity.

Glaring into his face, I asked, "Is this the normal way your patients get their tub baths?"

Mr. Kent looked up at me and gave me a crooked smile. "It's okay, nurse, I'm used to it all now. Still, as I told you yesterday, it's nice to meet someone who doesn't think it's the right way to look after us."

"I certainly don't agree with what's happening here. You deserve much better than this."

The attendant had not stopped what he was doing and I was getting wet from all the splashing. I stepped back and looked around for a towel.

"You'd better get yourself out of here." The orderly growled. "This isn't any of your business or concern. You needn't think you can do anything to change the way we've been doing things around here for years. Just get out, right now." He hollered. "Just leave us alone."

With my ire raised over this man's poor attitude, I turned and marched out of the tub-room. I was determined to do something about what I had just witnessed.

Finding my instructor, I relayed all that I had seen. I told her how it was contrary to all that she was teaching us about patient's rights. She agreed with me.

After each work period on the ward was over, we had a conference session. During this time we would discuss any issues of incidents that had occurred while we were working. "Patients needs for privacy," was our major topic that day.   It was unanimously agreed that everyone has the right to be treated at all times with dignity and respect.

Together, as a class, we compiled a letter of protest to the hospital administration. For the remainder of our tour of duty on that ward, those aspects of patient care were much improved. This gave all of us a great deal of satisfaction as well as a sense of accomplishment. We might only have been students but we had been heard and we had succeeded in getting a wrong reversed.

The Difficult Role

A young woman, named Helen, was admitted to the respiratory floor. She had suddenly experienced a lot of difficulty with breathing. Before her admission, she had been relatively healthy. Helen didn't know why this was now happening to her. She held the oxygen mask tightly on her pale, anxious face as she tried to get air.

Helen's husband was a successful businessman. They were living abroad and had come back to Canada to visit with their two children who were attending school here. It was the sudden onset of this lady's symptoms that mystified the specialists.

The plan was to conduct several investigative procedures in the hope that the reason for this lady's distress could be found. The doctor in charge was confident that they would be able to help her.

My job was to assist in some of her care. Helen was a charming young woman. Her graciousness, even though she was having major problems breathing, made us feel she appreciated the care we were providing.

Helen's call bell was frantically ringing. Her primary nurse was busy so I went in to see what she needed. The small features covered by the oxygen mask stared fearfully at me. Beads of perspiration had flattened her short blonde hair and the heavy, rale sounds of her breathing filled the air. I didn't need anyone to tell me, I could see, that this lady was very ill.

Helen clamped her hand over mine when I ventured to lift the mask of her face so she could tell me what she wanted. I nodded and left it on while she wrote on a sheet of paper why she'd called for help. More air please. I have to get more air.

As I was not sure of the strength or amount of oxygen that she was getting I gently touched her shoulder. "I'm just going to check with your nurse what your oxygen should be set at. I'll be right back."

After I quickly found the nurse who was caring for Helen, I relayed the concerns that the patient had and what I had observed while with her. "I'll go at once and see her, " the nurse told me.

"Have they been able to make a diagnosis as yet?"

Helen's nurse shook her head. "I hope that they come up with one soon. This lady is getting very tired." She hurried off towards her patient's room while I made my way back to the desk.

The Specialist who headed the respiratory team was at the desk. He looked up from studying a chart as I appeared at his side.

"I've just come out of your patient's room down the north hall. You know she's in a great deal of distress. Her breathing sounds absolutely awful."

He peered at me over the top of his glasses, a habit he often displayed. "I'm not surprised that she's experiencing major problems with her breathing. I'm sad to say this lady has a huge tumor, which keeps cutting, off her air supply. The worse thing is there's nothing we or anyone else can do to help her."

"I'm so sorry to hear that." I said. "How are you going to tell her?"

"Well!" He removed his glasses. "I will have to go and tell her soon, but I'm going to wait until her husband comes in. Then she'll have someone to give her the support she's going to need when she hears what I have to say."

As I had always held this Doctor in high regard knowing that he genuinely cared for his patients, I could sense he was saddened by what he had to do. I watched him with concern as he moved slowly away from the nurse's station.

The following day I saw the specialist talking with Helen's husband. His face blanched and became distorted with grief as he heard the bad news. The Doctor quietly waited until the man calmed down. They then walked together down the hall.

Shortly thereafter, I saw the specialist come out of the room alone. As he moved up the hallway his large frame was stooped over. His face was unsmiling and grim.

As he came towards the desk, I felt some of his grief at what he had just had to do. Respecting this I never spoke but just nodded to him as he passed by the nurse's station.

Helen died the next day. Although death was a frequent visitor on this unit there was a feeling of immense sorrow amongst most of the staff as well as the medical team about this lady's passing. This was one of those instances when we all learned what it is to feel helpless when faced with a problem that was inevitable.

Another Way to Communicate

This is going to be very difficult. I smiled at the middle-aged woman seated on the bed. The volunteer had told me that Mrs.Veroot spoke little English. She did speak a lot of Dutch, which I didn't speak or understand. Yes, I thought, getting her history is certainly going to be a challenge.

"Hello," I said. I pointed to myself. "I'm your nurse and I have to do your admission."

Mrs.Veroot smiled and nodded. "So sorry, so sorry, English no so good."

"That's okay." I said."Somehow or other we will manage. I patted her arm and pointed to the scales, where I wanted her to stand. She did as I requested.

She was being admitted to the ward for an assessment of an ophthalmology condition. I noticed that she frequently rubbed her right eye, which looked reddened and sore.

I pointed to her eye, and grimaced. "Your eye, it pains you?" I asked her. She frowned, and shook her head. I had no idea if she had understood what I had been trying to convey by all my facial contortions. Nevertheless, she was my patient, and I knew that I would have to proceed the best way I could to get all of her information documented.

"So sorry.....So sorry," she said, as she hung her head down. "Is no goot. No goot!"

"It's alright." I smiled, and patted her arm. She peered at me. "It really is."

She rubbed at her eye again, and I certainly did not need her to tell me that it hurt. The drawn expression that passed across her face whenever she touched it was enough.

With a lot of mime, and a great deal of nodding and shaking of both of our heads, I finally had all of Mrs.Veroot's paperwork completed. As I left her room, I wondered how the doctor from the eye service was going to do his admission. I thought it best to forewarn him of the language problem. When I relayed this information to him, he thanked me.

A few days later, the specialist approached me while I was at the nurses' station. "Do you have Mrs.Veroot today as a patient?" he asked.

I nodded. "Yes, I do."

"Do you speak any Dutch?"

I shook my head. "No, I'm sorry I don't."

"That's too bad," he muttered.

"Yes," I said, "It would have made it a lot easier if I did, but we've been managing okay up to now, without verbally saying very much."

"Well, that's fine then," he said. "Perhaps, you could go in right now and see her. She's very upset about her diagnosis."

"What did her test show?" I asked.

He pursed his lips together before answering. "They were not good. This lady is going to have to have that right eye of hers removed, and it needs to be done soon."

I could only imagine how this woman must have been feeling, knowing how I would react to such news myself. "I'll go in at once," I said.

When I walked into her room everything about her posture indicated someone in a great deal of distress. Mrs.Veroot sat slumped in the middle of the bed sobbing, and rocking backward and forward. I walked over to her and placed my arm around her shoulders. She looked at me with her tear-stained face and gave a deep heart-wrenching sigh.

I wanted to let her know that I empathized with her, and I wanted to be able to tell her in some other way than just hand signals and a few odd words of English. The problem was how to do that.

Then I spotted her Bible on her bedside table. Although it was printed in Dutch, I picked it up.

Mrs.Veroot watched me as I leafed through the pages. I finally found the section I wanted. In the book of Ecclesiastics, there is a passage that has given me much comfort when I needed it. I hoped that it would ease some of my patient's pain, and let her know that I understood she felt. I pointed to Chapter 3 and motioned to her to read it. The passage begins - "For everything there is a season, and a time for every matter under Heaven..."

She sat quietly looking at the page. Her tears gradually subsided, and she turned towards me and nodded.

I inclined my head back at her. As I was about to leave, Mrs.Veroot grabbed hold of me and hugged me. We had not said a word during this short exchange, but by using the help of God's word, I had found a way to communicate with her.

The Culprit was what

Nurses and doctors are occasionally able to lighten up and do enjoy a good laugh as well as a funny joke. If the situations were related to them personally this would create even more amusement.

On the cardiovascular-respiratory unit, a visiting physician noticed that the majority of the younger married staff were pregnant. This caused some of the older members working on that floor to wonder jokingly if there might be an inanimate object which could be the culprit. This idea turned into a conviction when it was learned that not only was there a rash of expecting mothers working on that unit but also several of the young doctor's wives were in the family way.

It was agreed there had to be an illogical explanation for this phenomenon. The task we set ourselves was to try and track down the guilty party. Amid much laughter there was several suggestions put forth that could have caused this unusual situation.

Maybe it was related to the drinking water? Because some of the younger doctors didn't take any liquid refreshment of any kind while working on the floor, this was ruled out. Then one wag suggested maybe a patient had impregnated a box of chocolates with hormones and this might have got everyone going. As someone who enjoyed taking a sweet with the best of them I pooh-poohed this theory. " Why had I been able to escape this sudden display of fertility?"

I was then reminded, in a kind way, "that I had done my bit many years earlier for the propagation of the species by having had and raised two fine children. I was now therefore, ruled immune and safe."

I couldn't disagree with that, yet having all these people around who were beginning to show definite signs of motherhood made getting any help with heavy patients, who needed to be lifted and moved, very difficult. Those of us who hadn't succumbed to the pregnancy trend tried hard not to have to go to those who had for any additional assistance. Most of us older members felt that these mums-in-waiting should be getting a rest in the afternoons, not running around caring for others on a busy ward.

However, I digress. We still had to find out what or who was the guilty party. As mentioned there were a lot of good-natured ribbing and weirder ideas about the cause of the present situation on this unit.

We had considered the water as well as a possible tampering with treats but these suggestions were quickly discarded. Then by a lucky coincidence and the keen imagination of a physiotherapist it was agreed that it had to be one of the chairs in the nurse's station. It had to be one of them because everyone at some time or other sat down to chart, write orders or whatever. Now the hypothesis was proposed, all that remained for us to do was to zero in on the actual culprit.

Again this gave us many laughs but finally there was a chair picked and labeled as the perpetrator. For several months that particular piece of furniture was avoided like the plague.

Also funny was the fact, that once they heard the reason for its banishment, even people who were infrequent visitors to that unit would not sit in that chair. Even if it meant that they had to stand, they preferred to do that. As soon as the rash of pregnancies had gone to full term and the babies all safely delivered it was reprieved. To my knowledge, this piece of furniture was never again involved in any further indiscretions.

The Accomplishment

"Let me out of here." The elderly woman snarled fiercely. "If you don't help me get up I'm going to call the police." Jessie wagged a small finger in front of my face. "You'd better do as I say, " she added. "Are you listening to me?"

Jessie was a small wiry, lady in her early eighties and because of problems with her balance, she was unable to walk. We had told her this many times, but still she would persist in her demands to be helped out of her chair.

"Don't you look at me like that." She tried to reach my hand, which I'd placed on her shoulder.

"You're just like the rest of them, so don't be trying to get around me. I know what you're all like."

"Jessie, " I whispered. "There's nothing that I'd enjoy more than to see you get up out of this chair, but you would fall and could break something."

"I most certainly would not, " she yelled. "You are just saying that. You don't care one bit about my feelings." Her voice trembled, and tears began to trickle down her cross features.

"Oh! Jessie that's not true and you know it. But, if you're sure this is what you want to do I'll get another nurse to help me, and we'll see if we can get you up."

The tears stopped as quickly as they had begun. My hand was given a rough squeeze. The oval, lined face now grinned at me.

Coming out of Jesse's room I made my way to the nurse's station. Mid-morning was a busy time, and I knew it would be difficult to get someone to assist me.

The head nurse was sitting at her desk, engrossed in paper work. "Excuse me." I said softly, trying to get her attention.

50

"What is it? Can't you see I'm busy?"

"I've promised Jessie Williams, that I'll try and get her up out of her chair." I said. "However, I need someone to help me as I can't do it alone."

"You've done what?" She muttered crossly. "Jessie hasn't stood up for months. And, even if she could we have quite enough to do without catering to every demand that patients make." She shooed me way with her hands.

"I strongly suggest, "she said curtly, "that you get on with your other work and forget this ridiculous idea. Now go away and leave me alone. I haven't got time for this."

It was useless saying anything else to her. But, what was I going to tell Jessie? I'd made her a promise.

In a long term, facility there is not a lot of spare time for extra tasks. Regardless, I was determined that somehow I was going to give my patient what she wanted.

I carried on with the rest of my assignment, and at odd intervals I popped into Jesse's room to let her know I hadn't forgotten her.

"You're really going to help me stand up?" She asked several times. "Yes I am, Jessie, " I assured her. "But you need to be patient for a little while longer until I get finished."

"You're not lying. Are you?" She'd ask repeatedly.
I'd shake my head and say, "No Jessie I'm not."

Finally, I had the time to go and see her. First of all I had to find another nurse to give me a hand.

Nancy quickly agreed to assist me. When we entered Jesse's room, it appeared that she was having a sleep.

"Perhaps we should leave her and come back later, " Nancy whispered.

"Oh! No you don't, "Jessie said. She sat bolt upright in her chair. "I wasn't sleeping. I'm all ready for you. I've been waiting here for hours. "Her blue eyes gleamed with excitement and anticipation.

"Okay, how are we going to do this?" Nancy said. "Do you think we'll need to get the Hoyer lift?"

"There's no way that I'll agree to that." Jesse's small features glared crossly. "I'm not getting lifted up in that horrible contraption. You promised me that you'd help me to stand on my own two feet, and that's what I want to do."

"Well, that's all well and good." Nancy looked anxiously at me. "But how long is it since she has actually stood up?"

"I'm not sure." I said. "Anyway, we'll give it our best shot because that's what I've promised. We're both strong and she isn't very big or heavy so it shouldn't be too difficult."

"If you stand behind her, Nancy, I think we'll be able to manage just fine."

I positioned myself in front of Jessie and told her she would have to clasp her hands behind my head once I bent down towards her. Her face was close-up in front of mine, and the big smile on it convinced me we were doing the right thing.

Her hands were fastened behind my head as we asked her if she was ready. "Oh yes indeed, I'm all ready." She chuckled with glee.

"Okay, " I told her. "On the count of three I'll grip your knees with mine and Nancy will hang onto your back."

On the third count I locked Jesse's knees with my own and brought her to an upright position. Her legs wobbled a bit, but we were able to keep her standing for a few minutes. Just before I put her back in her chair she planted a large sloppy kiss on my cheek, and whispered, "Thank-you. Thank-you, thank-you.... so much."

"I told you I could do it. Didn't I. Didn't I?" Jessie could barely contain her happiness. "And I really did."

Placing my arm gently around her shoulders, I acknowledged that she had indeed stood up, even if it had been for a fleeting moment.

"Now Jessie," I said. "We have to get back to the rest of our patients. Is there anything else you need before we leave?"

"No, there's nothing else I want, thank-you. "She gave a long sigh. "I stood up. I really stood up, and that's all I wanted to do."

Nancy and I quietly walked out of her room leaving behind one contented lady. From then onward Jessie was less demanding and easier to please. Whenever she had the opportunity she'd remind us of what she had been able to do that day. For some people this achievement likely wouldn't mean much but for this elderly woman it was a major accomplishment. I was glad to have been there to help her realize it.

A Cry from the Heart

His gaunt face looked as pale as the sheet that covered him. His sunken eyes, rimmed with dark circles, flickered with a faint smile of recognition.

Mr. Campbell had been a policeman most of his working life. Because of his deteriorating health his wife hadn't been able to manage him at home so he was now under our care. He had multiple health problems. The major one was a very poor circulatory system, and due to this all of his body had started to break down.

This elderly man hated to be in the in hospital. "I don't like being here, "he frequently said. But, often he would also add, "I wish my life was over and done with"

Despite the despondency over his situation, Mr. Campbell was an easy person to look after. Although he was what we called, "a heavy patient, "and the staff had to provide total care for him, he wasn't at all a demanding person. He was always grateful for the nursing we provided, and would often graciously tell us so.

Entering his room, after a period of absence, I smiled.

"So Mr. Campbell, " I said." How have you been?"

"Just about the same, I guess. I'm still here anyhow."

"Yes, you are Mr. Campbell, " I said trying to build him up with some cheer and a smile. "In addition, you get to have me as your nurse for the next four weeks. What do you say to that?"

"That's fine with me." He looked pensive as he added, "You at least always seem to know how I'm feeling and understand why I feel sad. I know for some people that is not easy. They just think I should be glad to be alive, but I'm not." His voice trembled, and his brown eyes mirrored his misery. I gently touched him on the cheek.

I had read his history from the chart, and knew something of his background. As well as a busy working life, he had been an active man in his community, volunteering and assisting others. His wife's decision to place him in a chronic institution had been in part because she wanted to continue with her own career. She had never, even though she'd been called many times, returned to see her husband.

He had no other family, and his few friends, for whatever reason, had stopped coming in to see him. He was all alone.

When a patient reaches the stage where all they want to do is die, and that is all they talk about, it can be very hard on the nursing staff. I invariably found it was easier when that person held some belief in a spiritual aspect of life. It always helped because it seemed to give them some meaning for their suffering.

Mr. Campbell didn't have that coping tool as he often said, "Once this life is over with that's it, there's absolutely nothing else."

It is tempting at times to want to try to change such people's philosophy, but that is not in a nurse's job description. My primary role was to care for this man to the best of my ability and to ensure he was kept as comfortable as possible.

However, it certainly was not easy. This man's body was in a dreadful condition. When we went to reposition him in bed there was barely anywhere on his tall frame that we could touch, without the fear of further damaging his paper-thin skin.

Nevertheless, what I clearly remember about him is what he asked me to do, while I was one day attending to him. I had removed the pillows from under his head and along with another nurse was preparing to turn him.

Mr. Campbell quietly, firmly, but out of character, said, " Just put the pillow over my face girls. That's all it'll take. Then I'll go to sleep and that will be that."

I have never forgotten those heart-wrenching words. To me they echoed all his hurting body and the immense mental sorrow he felt.

My voice choked. "You know we could never do a thing as that." He had closed his eyes and made no verbal response, but his body shook when we turned him.

My peer spoke brusquely. "That's quite enough of that Mr. Campbell. You know you shouldn't have said that to us, and we don't want to hear you repeating it ever again."

"Aren't you being a bit hard on him, " I said, as we finished getting him settled.

"I don't like hearing that from any patient, " she muttered. "And he should know better than that. Wasn't he once a policeman?"

In retrospect, she was probably right. But, at the time all I could think of was that this poor man sorely needed some major intervention to manage the way he was feeling.

"I'm sure that he knows that we couldn't that, " I said to her. "But we should not chastise him. We need to look for a way where we can best help him."

"Well you do what you want, " she grumbled. "I'm going to let the supervisor know about this."

"He is my patient, " I said. "Moreover, I am responsible for him. I'll see that the supervisor is informed, and I'd appreciate it if you don't say anything to her or anyone else about all of this."

She shrugged her shoulders as she made her way to the door. "I suppose that's okay but just see that you do tell her."

All this time Mr. Campbell had been lying still and saying nothing. Now I turned back to him and stood by his bedside.

"The other nurse is right you know. I will have to inform the supervisor about this but only because we want to help you. Perhaps the Doctors need to increase your pain medication or give you a mood elevating drug so you won't be so depressed."

Mr. Campbell peered up at me. His face was full of anguish. "I'm truly sorry nurse, I should never have said that to you. I've only made things really awkward for you." His voice choked. His thin emaciated hands grasped the covers. I gently placed my hands over his. "It's alright, I understand, really I do. Now, if you'll just excuse me, I'm going to go and get you the help you desperately need."

When I reported all this to my supervisor, she immediately contacted the institution Doctor on-call. Mr. Campbell had his medication increased and he had something to help ease his despondency. He slept more but appeared to be in a much better frame of mind.

Neither he nor I spoke of this incident again. I was just gratified that he was able to enjoy the last few days of his life more comfortably, until one morning his struggle with life quietly ended.

Ridden with Guilt

"I don't know how I'm ever going to be able to face my wife," Mr.Rocco said dejectedly. His swarthy complexion looked paler than I remembered, and appeared drawn and pinched. I knew that the medical team had told him his diagnosis, which could not have been easy for him to hear.

Mr.Rocco had been admitted to the ward because of some health concerns that his family doctor wanted to explore further. When I met him for the first time, I had thought he was a charming man. Now I was not sure how I felt about him.

Nurses are not supposed to harbor any ill will towards any patient. This might be fine in theory but it is sometimes difficult not to have unpleasant thoughts about a person. Although I felt sorry for the middle-aged man now sitting in front of me, I was also disgusted because of what he had done and the serious implications to his family. Nevertheless he was in my care and that took priority over everything else.

I looked into his worried face. "How are you going to tell your wife about your problem?" I asked.

"It's not going to be easy for me," he murmured. "Telling my wife what I've got."

Not easy for you, I thought. It is going to be devastating for her.

I knew from the information he had given me earlier that he had been married for twenty years. He had two sons and one daughter. Mr.Rocco had even proudly shown me some photos he had of them all. It had seemed at the time that he thought a lot of his family and that they were very important to him.

So why would he have done this? I couldn't help thinking what a tragedy this had become. Yet, I silently reasoned he must have realized there were risks before he had himself

58

involved in such promiscuous act. My thoughts about him were mixed.

By his agitated state, however, I could see that this man did not need me to pass judgement on him as he already had done that to himself. What he needed was my support.

Bending closer to him, I said. "Maybe you need someone with you when you talk to your wife? I can easily arrange something with the social service department if you'd like that?"

He shook his head several times. "No! No! No!" he firmly replied. "My wife would get very upset if a lot of strangers knew about our personal affairs."

"I never meant to do anyone any harm," he added softly. "I've never ever done anything like that before. How could such a thing have happened with only the one time?"

"What did you know about the person that you had this encounter with?" I asked.

He turned away from me and mumbled something.

"I'm sorry I didn't hear what you just said there. Could you repeat it for me."

Anguish was etched into his face and he appeared a lot older than his early fifties. He slowly turned back towards me. "I knew absolutely nothing about that person. I only did it because my wife was away visiting her relatives in Italy, and my buddies thought it would be a great lark. Now I'm going to suffer the rest of my life because of it."

"Yes,"I said gently,"you're right, it isn't going to be easy for you. But, although you're the one who's been diagnosed as HIV positive what do you think its going to do to your wife and your family when they find out?"

Then Mr.Rocco began to sob. His well-rounded body shook and the tears welled and spilled down onto his navy colored shirt. It was sad to see this man upset and crying so hard.

I placed my hand lightly on his shoulder. "What can I do to help?"

"There's nothing you or anyone else can do for me," he gulped." I just wish I could turn back the clock and none of this would have happened."

"I do understand," I said. "Unfortunately it has happened, and now you have got to find a way to explain it all to your loved ones."

He was still crying and I sensed from this that my patient was not sure how he was going to be able to face them. It was not a pleasant situation for anyone to have to face and I genuinely wanted to help him.

I waited until he had calmed down before speaking to him again. It was obvious that when he talked to his wife he was going to need someone with him.

In the acute care institution we were fortunate to have several services that provided this kind of support. I would need his consent before I could call any of them.

"Look," I patted his arm. "I think this is going to be way too difficult for you when you tell your wife what you've got, and the tests she will need to undergo. Suppose instead of a social worker I get someone from the chaplain's office to come and be with you?"

He sat quietly for several moments as if he was thinking this over. Nodding he answered." Yes, that might be all right. I just know, nurse, I cannot do this on my own."

So it's what was arranged. I talked first with a clergy representative and he was present when Mr.Rocco's wife was told of her husband's condition.

I can still see her as she came out of her husband's room accompanied by the minister. She had been crying, but I was glad she at least knew her husband's problem.

When he was finally discharged, this lady came to the desk and thanked me for having cared for her husband. He sat quietly in a wheelchair waiting to be taken home. He wasn't at all like the outgoing, cheerful man that I had first admitted. Although he firmly shook my hand, his whole demeanor was that of a tragic man. In that brief instant, I felt a great sadness for all the Rocco family, knowing that their lives had been changed so dramatically.

On his Own Terms

"If you think you're going to get me out of this bed, " Mr. Reid's elderly face glowered, "You've got another think coming. I'm not getting up for you or anybody else." He held the blankets firmly up around his chin.

"That's just fine with me. I'm your nurse today and as far as I'm concerned you can stay right where you are."

His grey, bushy brows rose in astonishment. "Well that's a switch. Usually I'm told I've got to get up, and that's that. The other nurses didn't give me a choice."

I smiled. "Well today you have."

Before meeting Mr. Reid, I'd been told that he refused to cooperate with any rehab program that was presented to him. Even though he wasn't in any immediate danger of having a relapse from his heart problems he was emphatic he was dying. I hadn't yet had him as a patient so I needed to find out from him just what he thought was happening. Many of the staff had said, he was just plain cantankerous and difficult, and if I could get him to change it'd be a miracle.

Not being one to shy away from a challenge I had offered to take him on. Looking now at his negative body language, I was not sure how I was going to even be able to give him a bath. Surprisingly, when I bathed him he didn't seem to mind a bit. He offered me an arm or leg as I proceeded through his care but flatly refused to talk.

I persisted in my attempts to get him to speak. "I've heard you used to be fond of playing golf. It's a game that I've never tried myself. How difficult is it?"

Mr. Reid scowled. He muttered something under his breath but I couldn't make out what he was saying.

"I believe you said something. I'm sorry but because you spoke so low I didn't understand what it was."

"Yes I do, or did, enjoy a game of golf." He muttered. "But I'll never again be able to play so quit talking about it."

"I don't believe that." I said.

"What don't you believe?" Mr. Reid bellowed.

"That you'll never again be able to play a round of golf."

"I'm dying. Don't you people understand? Here I thought you might be different, but you're just like all the rest of them."

I'd finished his morning ablutions, and before starting on anything else I stood quietly looking down into the angry, reddened face of this old gentleman.

"Mr. Reid," I said softly. "You're not in any immediate danger of dying. In fact all of your test results show your condition as being stable. The problem, sir, is that you have to want to get better and want to go home, and that is something that only you can decide upon. The decision is completely in your hands."

"You're saying I'm making this all up. I know how I feel. You don't."

"Well, I think I'll let you have a rest for now. That will also give you some time to think about what I have told you. I'll come back later and do your bed."

Going back to the nurse's station, I was greeted by a few of my peers grinning at me. One of them, Nancy, asked, "Well how did you make out with him? Bet you didn't get him out of his bed."

I smiled back at them. "No I didn't get him up because I gave him a choice today, but I think I've also given him something to think about."

"Told you it would take a miracle to change that old curmudgeon." Nancy chuckled to herself, as she moved away from the desk.

As I busied myself looking through my patient's charts I wondered if maybe she was right. It was going to take a miracle to get Mr. Reid to change his attitude.

I did not get anywhere that day with trying to change Mr. Reid negative behavior. The following day, however, using the same tactics and some extra coaxing I saw some positive action from him.

On returning to his room mid-morning I was amazed to find him out of his bed. He was sitting in his chair gazing out of the window.

"It's lovely outside at this time of the year isn't it, Mr. Reid?"

For a minute he didn't respond. Then he turned to face me. "When I was a young man I hated this time of the year. I was raised on a farm and the spring was always such a busy season. Now I've come to realize it's a beautiful one. I'm afraid I'm not going to see many more."

"Mr. Reid, " I said gently. "No one knows from one day to the next how many days we have to enjoy anything. The scriptures tell us, not to worry about tomorrow but to only concern ourselves in living today. I don't know about you but that's really all I'm able to do."

"Yeah! Yeah! That's all very well for the scriptures to say that, but what about someone like me with a serious health condition?"

"What about you? The fact you have got yourself up today is a big start. It's several days since you've done that and that tells me you really would like to get active again.

"I guess. He smiled. "But what will happen tomorrow?"

I laughed, and shook my head. "If I knew that I could make my living telling fortunes. As I've told you there's not a person alive who knows what's in store for them tomorrow. So why don't we just concentrate on each day as it comes."

"Well, all right then." He said, grinning. "Still if I'm going to get back home it's going to take a lot of work. My legs still feel weak and I've lost some weight as well."

"Suppose," I said, "we make up a wall chart. Each day we can then monitor your progress and you'll have something that'll show you how you're doing. This will also give all your nurses a basic plan of your daily care."

"And they will all follow it?"

"Most certainly. I'll put a note in your chart and Kardex that it's on the wall in your room, and what we've agreed to do."

Mr. Reid nodded. "Yes! I like the sound of that. Can I choose how much I do each day?"

"I think that'll be okay." I said. "As long as you remember we want to get you strong enough so you can eventually go home. And also get to go and play another round of golf."

It took the best part of two weeks to get this man fit enough to be discharged. Once he had his list up in his room and the staff kept him focused on achieving what he'd planned for each day he became a totally different person. His whole attitude changed from that of being a difficult, crotchety patient to one eager to get out of hospital and resume enjoying his life.

On his discharge day, Mr. Reid was not my patient. Still when he came up to the desk accompanied by one of his sons he beckoned to me. Grabbing hold of my hand he gave it a friendly squeeze.

Turning to his son he said, "This nurse is the one who made me see I had to want to get better. She helped me so much I will always be indebted to her.

"Well dad, she certainly did a good job with you. You're a changed man from the one that you were a couple of weeks ago."

"Mr. Reid." I let go of his hand, " I didn't do it all on my own. The other staff members on the floor also helped."

"Yeah yeah, " he saucily winked, " but you made out my work schedule and it was you who urged me on. You deserve a lot of credit for that."

"Well I'm just pleased that everything has turned out so well for you. Now when you come back to the clinic I expect to hear you've been out pushing that little white ball around your favorite course."

On his visit to the out patient clinic he left me a present which I was very reluctant to accept. Getting personal gifts isn't something hospital administration encourages. Nevertheless, the Chief of Staff on that particular ward made me take the toiletry travel case. He said that I deserved it. Mr. Reid was insistent that I should have it, especially as I'd been right all along and he had indeed got to again play a round of golf."

Therefore, I cheerfully accepted it. Now every time I use it this old gentleman's face always flashes through my memory. His gift is another reminder of how fulfilling nursing was for me.

Courage Facing Adversity

Some people throughout their lives never know what it means to struggle. Matthew wasn't so fortunate. He had been born with Cystic Fibrosis, which meant he had a constant battle with this pernicious opponent.

Matthew spent a lot of time on the respiratory unit. He knew most of us by our first names as well as a great deal about our personal lives; he was more as an extended member of each of our own families. That happened sometimes on that unit, especially if the individual was frequently admitted because of their health problem.

I had only been working on that ward for a few weeks when he was admitted for his usual physical assessment. Going into his room I found a tall, slightly built young man busily getting himself settled in. He greeted me with a charming smile.

"Ah!' he said, "you must be the new person I've been hearing so much about."

"Mm! I don't know if I like the sound of that, " I muttered. " What have you been told?"

He laughed loudly. "Oh! Nothing bad I assure you. It was mainly about your British accent."

I smiled back at him. "Yes it's something I can't easily disguise. I'm guess I'm just stuck with it."

"Well it's really very nice, " he added. And, it's not something you should try to hide."

Thanking him for the compliment, I proceeded to get his admission documents filled out. I was fascinated to learn that although he was only In his mid-twenties he had graduated from University and was also a very successful businessman.

"It's been hard at times, " he told me, " especially when this condition I've got really flares up. But I've tried my best not to let it beat me."

"You've done more, it seems, than a lot of people take their whole lives to do." I said. "That's quite an achievement, and one you can be proud of."

He flashed me another, broad smile. "You're very kind to say that."

"Well Matthew, I honestly meant it." I said as I moved towards the door. "See you later."

While he was a patient on the ward, and if he was able, he would be out socializing with staff or trying to aid the other patients. He was a warm, personable young man and it was hard seeing him suffer so much. He always tried to remain cheerful even when he was gasping for every breath.

He would constantly push his own problems aside and be concerned more about us or some other patient's welfare. Matthew was always ready to assist us in any way if he thought he could be of some help.

The only time I ever saw him show any brusqueness about his illness was when a young man came to see him about investments. I happened to be in his room and I heard him suggest that it was best to go for long term projects. Then he angrily muttered, " It's something I can't do. I'm not going to be around long enough."

This outburst surprised me, and yet I understood how frustrated he must have been feeling. It couldn't have been easy for him seeing someone about the same age as himself in such robust health. I also felt sorry for the young man because he did not seem to know what to say or do.

Nevertheless, he soon put the young man at ease by quickly apologizing. "I'm sorry I said that." Matthew said, looking embarrassed. " I'm usually not so insensitive." He then offered his visitor a hand to seal his expression of regret. When I left them they were again poring over the piles of papers, and deep in conversation.

As his condition deteriorated, his admissions became more frequent. All of the staff on the respiratory unit knew that it was only a matter of time, and this created a feeling of sadness on that unit. We were not just losing a patient that we had all got to know well, but he was also a friend.

Transplantation of another's lungs in the early 70's was not an option for patients with this disease. Today if Cystic Fibrosis is caught in its early stages that is a much stronger possibility. Matthew knew this but like the dozens of medications he had to take daily, the constant pummeling by physiotherapists to remove the sticky mucus from his lungs, he stoically accepted this reality too.

When he finally became bed-ridden and every breath wheezed and rattled, he still smiled and thanked us for his care. His warm, gentle personality stayed with him to the end.

He had Morphine to ease some of his agitation and the extreme pain. Finally, his long struggle ended one late afternoon when his life peacefully ended.

Matthews's brave battle with his disease, and his valiant struggle to live life well, will always remain with me. I believe it was a beautiful example of human courage, and strength, in the face of extreme adversity.

Unconditional Love

The white-haired man placed his arm around the plump elderly woman sitting in the chair. "Nurse, this is my dear wife Alice." He leant over and lovingly kissed her lined cheek.

"She wasn't always like this, " he added. "At one time she was a very successful businesswoman. She was very talented and clever. She could do all sorts of things."

Alice had made no movement or response to her husband's show of affection. She sat immobile, blankly staring ahead.

Alice's husband sat down in front of her and took hold of her hands. "You know nurse we have a son, but he doesn't come to see us anymore. He says, he can't stand seeing his mother like this."

Mr. Gold gave a deep sigh. "I wonder how he thinks I manage with it every day."

"That's one of the reasons why you're here." I smiled. Once the doctors have examined your wife and have a definite diagnosis, we can arrange some assistance for you. This will give you some respite in caring for your wife."

He caressed his wife's hands. "Some of my friends think I should put Alice into a home, " he murmured. "I just couldn't do that to her. She might not be able to recognize me but I certainly know who she is.

I nodded my head. "It's never an easy decision for anyone, " I said. "But there are some families who just can't manage, no matter how hard they try. Placing their loved one in a home is the only route they feel they can take."

Mr. Gold raised one of his wife's hands to his lips. "I don't know how they can even contemplate doing that. All I know is I never could."

"Your wife is fortunate right now that you're able to provide her with all the care she needs, " I said. "You know though it's going to get more difficult for you as time goes on."

He nodded. "Yes, I know that. I just wish sometimes, " he sighed, "that it was me that had been struck down with this terrible disease."

"Do you think it would have been any easier for her to look after you?"

Mr. Gold shook his head. "Probably not, but why did it have to happen to her of all people? She was such a vibrant woman. That's what attracted me to her in the first place. She was always busy doing something for someone or going some place."

When a person exhibited extreme forgetfulness in the early seventies, and was unresponsive to stimuli, it was often called senile dementia. Today it's more widely known as Alzheimer's Disease.

Nevertheless, whatever name it has, seeing a loved one struck down with this condition has to be one of the most difficult things anyone has to face. It's relentless, and there's no social level that escapes its grasp.

Mr. Gold smiled. "I think Alice knows who I am but she just isn't able to respond, that's all."

"Yes, maybe you're right Mr. Gold. I must say, Alice does look to be in good health other than her memory problem."

He gave a low chuckle. "I do make sure that she's well looked after. She's probably a lot healthier than I am myself right now."

Looking into this man's oval features, I could see that his statement held a lot of truth. Although he obviously adored his wife the toll on him was high, and it showed. Dark patches rimmed his brown eyes and his lined face was gaunt. I wondered how well he was attending to his own needs. I made a mental note to see that Mr. Gold health status was also assessed while we had his wife on our unit.

Alice allowed me to get her undressed so the doctors could do their preliminary examination. Her husband stayed in the room while I carried this out. He didn't physically interfere but kept up a constant one-sided conversation with her.

"You are going to be just fine my love, " he said. "I'll see that you have everything you need before I leave. You won't have to worry about a single thing."

Once I had Alice comfortably settled I turned to her husband." Mr. Gold, I would like to suggest that you take yourself down to the cafeteria and have something to eat. It'll soon be time for the supper trays to be delivered and I will see that she is fed."

He moved across to Alice and whispered something to her, and bent over and hugged her.

"You are right." He groaned, as he stood upright. "I could do with something to eat. You're sure that you'll see that my wife gets her supper?"

Propelling him to the door I said, " I promise. Now you go along and enjoy your own meal."

This caring, loving man was on the ward every day while his wife was a patient on our unit. He could be seen constantly talking to her which must have been heart breaking because Alice never gave any sign that she even heard him. With Mr. Gold, Alice's needs were always given priority over his own. To me the unconditional love that this man showered on his wife, who wasn't able to reciprocate, was both a beautiful but nonetheless a terrible sad thing to see. I was humbled by this mans unselfish commitment.

The Missing Link

"Have you got it girls?" Mr. Bradley anxiously asked. Janet and I looked across at each other and we both shook our heads.

"No sir not yet, " I said, smiling at the large man lying on the bed. "But, don't you worry we'll soon have you all fixed up."

Janet, the other nurse bent back over him. I stood ready to come to her assistance.

Just then, the thought struck me that nurses often said things that would not sound right if they were overheard. I also wondered what my husband would say if he could see what I was trying to do?

"There it is, " Janet yelled, "quick, get a hold of it."

Get a hold of what I thought. I couldn't see anything that was remotely big enough to make any sort of connection.

When Mr. Bradley had appeared on the ward his size had astonished many of us. He was well over six-feet tall and stocky built. I am only five feet tall with uniform shoes, so I felt like a midget along side of this man.

There had been some concern that he was not going to fit in a ward bed. Even though his feet extended slightly over the end-rail he had assured me, "It'll be fine nurse, just put an extra cover over my toes."

Nevertheless, this jovial man became quite distressed when I was doing his admission. "I have to get up a lot during the night to urinate," he told me. "That's when my breathing also gets bad. It's become a real nuisance for me."

"Not to worry," I said, "maybe we can fix you up with something at bed-time that will relieve both of those problems at the same time."

"That would be really great if you can." He beamed and looked calmer.

Taking into consideration this mans size I did not foresee anything that would interfere with this proposed plan. "Shouldn't be any trouble, "I said confidently" We'll get it all sorted out for you before we settle you down for the night."

Only two nurses were on the late shift, and we were kept busy getting everyone settled in his or her beds. Mr. Bradley frequently buzzed the desk and each time it was to ask the same question. "When are you going to get me fixed up so I can go to sleep?"

"Just as soon as we have a free moment, we'll be right in to see you," I repeatedly told him.

He always added, "You promise now, you won't forget."

"No Mr. Bradley," I said, trying to reassure him. "I've told you over and over again, we will do this for you. You've just got to give us time to get the rest of our work finished."

Now, here we were in his room trying very hard to accomplish something that was beginning to look nigh impossible.

Watching our repeated attempts he asked, " Have you got it in working order yet?"

Together Janet and I loudly exclaimed, with frustration. " No Mr. Bradley we haven't."

"There it is," my peer suddenly screamed. "For goodness sake, grab a hold of it."

Oh! My Lord, I thought, I can't believe this is happening. Two grown woman standing over the reclining figure of an elderly man struggling to apply a drainage device to his private appendage.

I made another vain attempt to do as I was told, but I was not fast enough.

"This is hopeless, " I said to Janet. "We'll just have to think of something else."

"Is it on yet girls?" Mr. Bradley, said anxiously.

I looked into this pleasant, elderly man's face and tried to sound unfazed. "No, I am sorry, we just couldn't get it attached, but don't worry I'll fix you up with something else. " I pulled the covers down over him. "It'll work just as well for you."

"I'm just a nuisance" he muttered. "I've caused you girls a lot of trouble, and all for nothing."

"No you haven't, " I said.

"Why couldn't you get that thing on?" he asked.

Not wanting to hurt this mans feeling, I sighed. "I don't really know sir. Anyhow, the thing is we do not want you to worry about it. By using an alternate plan, we were able to ensure that this pleasant man had a reasonably good nights sleep.

This incident, however, taught me an invaluable lesson: never think that a person's stature has any influence on the size of any other part of their anatomy.

Memories that made a Difference

"I can't stand much more of this, " Helen muttered through clenched teeth. "I've just got to have something for the pain."

Mary was a pleasant middle-aged lady who was on our ward with bone cancer. Her primary cancer had been in her breast, which had now spread. Her status was rated as "guarded". This was partly due to our inability to get her pain under control.

She was being given strong doses of analgesic along with a mood elevator but she was still not comfortable. The medical team did not want to increase either of these as they felt that her respiratory center would become depressed. She had also told them that she wanted to keep all her faculties alert for as long as it was possible.

Mary tossed and turned around in her bed as I tried to get her settled. Her small face looked pinched and drawn.

"Isn't they're anything else that can be done for this pain?"

"Yes, " I said, "there is something else we could try."

She quickly sat up, and grabbed hold of my arm. "What is it? Please tell me. I'm ready to try anything."

"The problem with this alternate form of therapy, " I said. "Is that it does not always work. If the patient really wants it to succeed then there's usually good results."

She squeezed my arm. "I am ready nurse. All I know is that I can't go on much longer like this."

"Okay. First, we need to have you either sitting or lying down. You pick which you prefer."

Mary chose to lie down. Once I had her settled as comfortably as possible I asked her to close her eyes. I dimmed the lights in her room and drew the drapes. She had been so busy listening to these instructions and following them out that she already appeared to me to be more relaxed.

"Now," I said. "What I want you to do is to think of a time, any time in your life, when you were happy. When you have that picture clear in your minds eye hold onto it."

Mary's face grimaced as she tried to recall something from her past. Then she looked up at me and smiled. "I've got it but I'm very young."

"That doesn't matter. Just keep a hold of it so you can relive that experience."

"I can see myself riding my pet pony." She laughed. "I loved him so much and we shared so many good times."

"That's very good Mary, " I whispered. " Keep that picture of you on your pony in front of your minds eye."

Mary was lying still as she recalled this period in her life. "What are you doing with him now?" I asked.

"We're out on the trail that used to run behind my parents farm. Lucky, that's what I called him. He always knew where to go. He was very clever."

"Is they're anything else about him that you remember?"

"Yes, " she said with a sigh. "How he enjoyed being groomed. How his coat would gleam and shine after I'd brushed him."

I let her lie quietly for a while as she captured all of this. Then touching her gently on her arm I said, "Now, I would like you to open up your eyes."

Mary was still smiling as she did as I had requested. "I haven't thought about Lucky in a long time, " she said. "That was very good nurse."

"How do you feel now?" I asked.

"Why you know something, " she sounded surprised, " the pain isn't as bad as it was. Why is that?"

I shook my head, " I can't honestly answer that. There are a lot of theories, about the body releasing certain chemicals into the blood when we do this, but it doesn't matter as long as it has given you some relief."

What I told Mary was the truth. I didn't know why recalling something pleasant could temporarily ease someone's pain. All

I did know was that with some patients it worked while with others it didn't.

After this initial experience, Mary was able to manage her pain problem better. Just by recalling those happy memories when she needed to, enabled her to help herself.

A Problem with Feet

"Now look at what you've done, " the large elderly man scolded, as I tried to get him to move away from his bed. This was his first attempt at walking since he had had his operation. "This isn't going to work, nurse. Look, my shoes are flip-flopping all over the place."

I met Mr. Ray for the first time, a week prior, when I had gone down to pick him up from the recovery room. He'd had kidney surgery and was still very groggy from the anesthetic.

Back in his room, I needed someone to assist me in getting him transferred from the stretcher to his bed. This I knew was not going to be easy. He was a heavy-set, built man.

However, before I was able to go and get help the head nurse of that unit appeared. She quickly offered her services to get my patient comfortably settled. I stood at the head of the stretcher while she positioned herself at the foot.

Removing the flannel cover that had been keeping him warm, Miss Short let out a loud shriek, "Oh! My goodness, Oh! My. Just look at his feet. Look at those dreadful, dreadful nails." From my vantagepoint, I could not see what had caused this extreme reaction from her.

"Take a good look at those feet, " Miss Short gasped. She pointed at Mr. Ray's extremities. Glancing at them, I saw they were large and bare.

I peered closer at them and gulped. This old gentleman's nails were the most monstrous looking things I had ever seen. They protruded at least four inches from the end of every toe. They were thick and looked more like horns. I couldn't Imagine how he had ever been able to walk with them.

"You see that you get them cut before he leaves here" Miss Short curtly ordered, as we moved Mr. Ray across into his bed.

I could not help wondering how she expected me to accomplish this, it seemed like an impossible task. Later that same day I brought my teacher in to look at my patient's neglected feet. "Good grief, " Mrs. Harrison spluttered. How did this man ever manage to walk with such terrible nails? He must have hobbled around everywhere."

Mr. Ray was now awake, and he sat up. "What's all the fuss over my feet?"

I stared at him in astonishment. "Have you seen the length of your toe-nails?"

He shook his head. "Now that's funny. How could I see them when I can't even get down to them."

"Well, they are really in a terrible state." I said. "And, I've been ordered to trim them."

I told my instructor about the strict command I had received from Miss Short. My teacher nodded. "Yes, I agree. I think that would be a good thing to do, and it will give you some valuable experience."

She carefully touched the end of each nail. "If you do it gradually; a little bit each day, that should work."

"Yeah, right." I thought.

Mrs. Harrison nodded again and smiled as she left me with this problem.

Mr. Ray was in no fit state that day to be interested in having anyone work on his feet, so I waited until the next day to begin this task.

Armed with a bottle of baby oil and some warm towels I went back to his room. He was quite interested in what I had planned. "What are you going to do with all that stuff?"

"Your nails have been neglected for a very long time." I muttered. "Before I can make any attempt to cut them I've got to get them softened."

"I know they need looking after," he said. "It's not that I haven't tried to trim them, but my belly, " he patted his large abdomen, and laughed, "it always got in the way."

"Yes, " I smiled, "I can see you might have a bit of a problem with that. But surely someone in your family could have done them for you?"

He shook his head. "Oh, no nurse. No! No! It just wouldn't be right asking either one of my daughters to do that."

"Why ever not?" I asked.

"I don't know, but it's not something I'd want either of them to do."

"You know, Mr. Ray, " I said, as I finished wrapping his feet, "If you have this kind of problem, I wonder how many more seniors there are in the community in the same situation?"

He frowned. "I'd have a quick guess there must be dozens of them."

It took several more treatments with warm towels before I could begin cutting his nails. Now, I was trying to get him to walk with them much shorter than when he had come into hospital.

"Look at what you've gone and done." He scolded. "My shoes are like giant boats."

As he tentatively stepped out, he added, with a chuckle. "It's okay, nurse, don't worry about it, I will get used to it. I'll just have to get me some smaller footwear."

He hooted with more laughter. "There's one thing for sure, though, I won't be making any more huge holes in my socks."

Before his discharge, his daughters brought him in some smaller shoes. When I told them why this was necessary they were amazed that their father had never let them know he needed that kind of help.

His comment, about dozens of others needing this type of care, later got me started on an additional career; providing foot care for seniors in their homes. Over the years I saw many other people's feet just as badly neglected, as I'd found this mans.

The Bare Necessity

Coming into hospital cannot be the nicest experience for anyone. Being admitted for the first time when you are in your senior years can be even more traumatic.

Mr. Jones appeared on the medical unit accompanied by a volunteer. It was obvious to us, who saw his arrival, that this was a very nervous man. He was panting and his large, square shaped face shone with beads of perspiration.

The head nurse provided him with a chair at the desk while I checked which room he was to occupy. She encouraged him to take slower breaths and gradually he was able to lower his respiration level. I saw, however, that he was biting his lower lip as well as looking anxiously around the ward. I needed to find out what was causing this man so much physical distress.

We walked slowly down to his room, with Mr. Jones tightly clutching my arm. Once I had him sitting comfortably in his room I drew a chair up and sat down beside him. I gave him a warm smile and gently patted his arm.

He suddenly blurted out, "This is the first time I've ever been in a hospital and I really don't like being here. It has a weird smell."

"Mr. Jones, " I said. "I do empathize with you. Coming into hospital isn't the nicest thing for any of us, but sometimes it's necessary when we are ill."

"But I'm not ill. I just have a bit of a problem with my breathing that's all."

"Yes I can see and hear that." He was noisily short of breath again.

"What's that odd whiff around here?" he wheezed. "It seems to be everywhere. It smells like some sort of strong disinfectant."

"I'm not sure what you mean about an odor. Perhaps I've got so used to it I don't notice it anymore."

His blue eyes crinkled at the corners as he grinned. "Or you might also have a problem with your snifter."

"You could be right there." I smiled. "Aside from that we'd better get started on your admission or I'll have other things to worry about."

"It didn't take too long to get all of his documentation completed although he frequently reminded me that this was the first time he had ever been in a hospital.

I tried to reassure him. I said, " that I knew this, and I'd make certain his doctor was told. Before leaving his room I gave him a hospital gown and suggested, "He change into it, as this would make it easier for his doctor to do the physical examination."

I had not been back at the desk for more than ten-minutes when there was a sudden ruckus in the area of Mr. Jones room. We heard a woman give a loud scream. This immediately made everyone at the desk jump up and rush to see what was happening.

Nearing his room, the screams from the elderly woman patient standing in the hallway became louder. The noise seemed to be, as we drew closer to that section, more as someone having a laughing fit.

What a sight met our eyes? Mr. Jones had put on the hospital gown as I had suggested but he had it on backwards. Being a portly gentleman, he wasn't able to keep the edges together so he was standing in his doorway with a lot of his flesh exposed. He was trying desperately to correct the problem, but it didn't matter how much he tugged at the gown nothing helped.

I quickly blocked him from the elderly, female patient's view and steered him back into his room.

"What kind of a stupid nightshirt do you call this." He spluttered crossly. "It barely covers anything."

Trying very hard not to laugh at his obvious exasperation, I smiled. "Yes, they probably do seem as an odd design, but there's a good reason for them being that way."

"Well I'm danged if I can figure it out." He plopped himself down on his bed, which only increased the gap between the edges of his gown.

"It's supposed to be worn the other way around." I said.

"That's ridiculous. If I put it on as you say my backside will be showing." He started to remove the offending garment.

"Whoa!." I grabbed hold of his arm and stopped his entire disrobing. "Any gown is better than having none on at all. What I'll do is give you another shirt and you can wear it over the one you've already got on, but the other way around."

"As long as my behind is all covered up. I don't like having that bare."

Helping him into his other gown I couldn't resist a chuckle as I said, "Well I think that having one's behind showing is maybe preferable to what you've just had all uncovered."

He gave a deep sigh. "Yes, perhaps you're right there. But you know I've never been in hospital before. I had no idea which way it was supposed to be worn."

Other than that one amusing incident, this pleasant gentleman's time spent on our ward was uneventful. Although it was the talk of the ward for a little while. In spite of that, I would like to think that he, sometime, has as much merriment as I have had in recalling his guileless goof with that gown.

In the Blink of an Eye

"I should have taken more care." The young woman on the stretcher wailed. "Now what am I going to do? Just look at the mess I'm in." She gently placed a hand over the eye patch that covered her left eye.

I did not know why she was so distraught. I did know she had come to the ward via the emergency department, which probably meant she had had an accident.

She sat upright and rocked back and forth, as she verbally attacked herself. "How could I have done something so stupid?" she sobbed. "I'm usually so careful. I'm always telling others how to avoid accidents, yet I didn't heed the warnings myself."

"Here," I said. "Let me help you into your bed. You will find it is a lot softer than the stretcher. That might help make you feel a bit better."

"Nothing is going to do that." She clenched her hands together.

"I'm sorry that you're feeling so badly." I said." However, I need to get your information, so you should know my name. Having told, I said. "And what are you called?"

"Idiot!" She spat out. "Just call me an fool because that's exactly what I am."

Glancing quickly at her armband, I saw that her name was Pat Baker. She wore a wedding band so I assumed she was married.

"You are being very hard on yourself. "Accidents happen all the time and often it's not because we've been careless or anything else, they just occur."

Mrs. Baker's small, pale, tear-stained face peered at me. The bulky dressing covering her left eye made her squint. Her right eye glared at me

"Nurse, I've already told you I'm an idiot, " she muttered. " How else can you explain away what I've gone and done to myself."

"Mrs. Baker," I gently touched one of her hands, " you're very upset right now, but we are all here to give you the help you need to get better."

She did not respond to my touch. Nevertheless, as her crying had eased I felt she had received some comfort from it.

"I will have to get you're chart completed, " I said. "But before I do that let me go to the desk and see when you last had anything for pain."

"I don't want anything for the pain. Tears spilled from her right eye. Pain means that my left eye is still all right." She again put her hand up to her bandaged eye.

"That's right nurse, isn't it?" she mumbled. "When you can feel pain in something it means it's alive. Doesn't it?"

"Mrs. Baker," I said. "I can see that you've injured one of your eyes. I can also see that it's been a terrible shock to you, but having pain in any body part isn't an indicator that it's fine. At the moment I don't know what kind of injury you've suffered."

She turned her back to me, and began to sob. "Oh, what am I going to do? I need both my eyes for my work, and I have a family to raise."

I was not getting anywhere with this patient. I needed to know the exact cause of her accident, and could only get that from her records. I would then be in a better position to provide her with the help she obviously needed.

Mrs. Baker turned back around and grabbed my arm. "Please, please tell me, that the doctors here will be able to save my damaged eye."

"The ophthalmology specialists here are very skilled, " I said. "They have successfully helped many, many patients. I'm sure that.............."

"Yes, yes, that's all well and good, " she muttered, "but can they save a badly injured eye like mine?"

"What did you do to it?" I asked.

My question made her again begin to cry. Taking a deep breath, she muttered. "I poked myself in the eye with a screwdriver. I was scraping some dried on paint off a window."

I winced. "Ouch!" I said.

"Yes, it dammed well hurt a lot when I did it." Her voice trembled.

"I can see why you are so upset, " I said. "Accidents like that, thank goodness, don't happen very often."

"Humph! She loudly exclaimed." I'd wager a bet that this has never happened to anyone else ever before."

I nodded. "Yes, you could be right." I patted her arm." Nevertheless, you are here now and the doctors, I know, will do everything they possibly can to save that eye. A lot, of course, depends on just how much damage you've done to it."

Mrs. Baker looked at me. This time her uncovered eye didn't display any anger; instead, it showed signs of her smiling. I smiled back at her.

She patted my hand. "You must think I'm a nut case for carrying on the way I've done?" she said.

"No! "I said. "I do understand. I would probably be feeling the same way had this happened to me."

"You're very kind, " she said, smiling at me. " I appreciate you letting me blow off steam."

Unfortunately, the doctors were unable to save Pat Baker's eye. She ended up having to have it removed.

This was a difficult thing for her, at first, to accept. I learned, however, she later found a way to use her accident as a measure to help others avoid doing the same sort of thing. She became a staunch advocate for accident prevention and spoke to many community groups on the subject.

Not Per the Book

The delivery room and the maternity wards were two of my favorite areas to work as a nurse. Working on the psychiatric unit was definitely, for me, the most difficult.

. It wasn't that I couldn't accept patients with mental disturbances were as ill as any with physical problems, but rather it was the form of treatment used to alleviate their illnesses that disturbed me.

It was during the Registered Nurse's training that I ran into trouble working in this area. What I did to help one of my patients was unconventional but at the time, I felt it was the only course of action to take.

Patty was in her early twenty's suffering from a behavioral condition. She was also the mother of a small daughter and permission had been given for her to have her child in with her.

Patty had been given a course of medications and counseling but wasn't responding to any of that. The first time I walked into her room I was appalled to see that she had placed her small daughter on the edge of the change table. The child could easily have toppled off and fallen on the floor. The baby's mother was sitting by the window reading a magazine and appeared to be totally unconcerned about the possible danger.

I had been told that all I was allowed to do with this patient was observe. Since I was not to interfere with what she did, I gritted my teeth and silently prayed for the baby's safety.

"Hello there, " I said, trying to make eye contact with Patty, "I see you have a lovely little girl. What do you call her?"

Patty showed no indication that she had heard me. I wanted very much to get a response from this young woman.

The potential danger that her child was in disturbed me greatly and I thought I just had to do something. I moved towards the change table and lifted the baby up.

Patty leapt up and snatched the baby from me. "Don't you touch her," she yelled. "Don't you dare touch her." Her cold anger made me cringe.

I backed away from her and trying hard to keep a normal voice, I said. "I didn't mean to upset you. It was just that your baby looked as if she was going to fall off the table that's all."

Patty's blue eyes glared at me. "Are you saying I don't know how to look after my own child?"

I shook my head, "No, no, that's not what I'm saying at all."

"Well that's alright then," she said softly. I was amazed how quickly her attitude had changed. She was now quiet and calm as she laid her baby on the bed.

It pleased me to see that the baby was on a much wider and safer surface. Patty returned to her seat by the window and resumed her reading.

One of the tasks assigned to me was to try to get this young woman to bathe something she had not done for over a week. Her unkempt appearance and body smell was becoming very unpleasant. The problem was how to accomplish this?

"Patty, " I said. Again, she made no evidence that she'd heard me.

"Patty, which would you prefer to have today a bath or a shower?" Still she ignored me.

"Look if you're concerned about your baby I can watch her for you, "I said.

The blonde tousled head looked up, "I don't want you touching my baby, do you hear?"

I nodded. "Yes I hear you."

"However, I won't touch her all I'll do is keep an eye on her while you're bathing. I'll call you right away if she needs anything."

"Well, I don't feel like bathing today, "she smirked, "so you won't have to concern yourself about watching her, will you?"

At that moment, the staff nurse came in with a bottle for the baby so I was not able to pursue this issue.

"I'll leave you to feed your own baby Patty, "the Registered Nurse said.

"You've got a student with you today. If you need help she can assist you." She placed the bottle beside the infant and walked out of the room.

Patty leisurely stood up. She causally picked up the bottle and began feeding her daughter. I froze when I observed the way she was doing this. She didn't give the baby any time to take a breath and I was afraid that the child would choke. With a lot of effort, I kept these fears to myself

Later that day, however, I vented my frustration to my instructor, "How am I supposed to help Patty if I'm only allowed to watch her?" I muttered.

"I wasn't able to get her to take a bath or a shower. And the way she feeds her baby really frightens me."

"Mrs. Stirling, "my instructor said kindly. "You're still in training." She smiled.

"Don't be so hard on yourself. You'll be surprised how quickly these patients can improve from day to day. I suggest you wait and see how your patient is doing when you come back tomorrow."

When I got home I tried to push all thoughts of Patty out of my mind but it was not easy. This young woman needed help but was I going to be the one to do it?

Going into her room the next day I found almost the identical situation that I had seen the previous day. The baby was lying on the change table in a position where she could fall off and her mother was sitting unconcernedly by the window.

That was when I blew my stack and I behaved in an unprofessional manner. First of all, I took the baby off the table. When Patty jumped and made a lunge for me I moved around the bed out of her reach. Laying the baby safely on the bed, I turned to face a very angry woman.

"Didn't I tell you yesterday not to touch my baby?" she screamed.

Patty stood immediately in front of me glaring into my face.

"Yes Patty, " I said, "you did tell me not to touch your child but I felt compelled to do something. She could have toppled onto the floor and I'm sure you wouldn't have wanted that to happen."

"Really, "she spat sarcastically. "Who made you such an authority on taking care of a baby?"

That was when I really lost it. I grabbed hold of her and gave her a thorough shaking. Immediately I realized what I had done. I could not believe my lapse of professional behavior. I was afraid for her and myself. She stared at me in utter amazement not saying a word.

Then in a low firm voice I said, "You will go into that bathroom, and take a shower. You will also wash your hair, and when you're done that, you will put on clean clothes. Do you hear me? As I was still holding tightly onto her, she just nodded.

After I had released her, Patty quietly gathered everything she needed and moved into the adjoining bathroom. She still hadn't said anything since I'd given her a shake and I wasn't sure if that was a good or a bad sign.

I checked to see that she was showering before sitting down beside the baby. Patty's little daughter wasn't any trouble. It was then I really began to worry about what I had done to her mother. How was I going to explain my conduct to my instructor?

Just then Patty came back into her room; a large towel wrapped around her slim body. Her blonde hair had been washed and she was briskly rubbing it dry. I quickly stood up and moved away from her baby.

She smiled at me, "That actually felt very good, " she said.

My thoughts were still in a state of confusion because of the way I had treated her. Also I knew that my actions were probably going to get me in deep trouble with my teacher and probably with the school authorities.

"I enjoyed that, " she said, running her fingers through her locks.

90

She turned to me, "Is my little girl alright?" She sat down beside her daughter, and lovingly caressed her.

"Yes Patty, your baby is just fine, " I said, "and I'm so pleased to see that you are feeling better."

Again, those blue eyes stared at me but this time they crinkled at the corners, by a smile. My heart was racing rapidly as I sent up a silent thank-you, thank-you that my unorthodox method of treatment had not misfired.

"I think I'll get dressed and then maybe take my little girl for a little walk. Can I do that nurse?"

"Yes, yes, by all means Patty. I think that's a lovely idea."

When the class met in the conference room at the end of our shift, my teacher zeroed in on the extraordinary change in my patient.

She looked inquiringly at me, "Why do you think this has happened?" she asked, raising her eyebrows.

"I'm not sure, " I said with a gulp, "but I have to tell you what I did today."

"Well let's all hear what you have to say, " her gentle tone only made my task harder.

"We're waiting." She smiled at me.

"Well it's like...mm...I had to do something. She wouldn't bathe and the way she looked after her baby made me ill."

"What do you mean you had to do something?" She pursed her lips. " What did you do?"

Taking a deep breath I blurted out, "I shook her. I gave her a good shaking."

For a few minutes, there was an uneasy hush in the room. Then in an angry voice my teacher yelled, "You did what? I can't believe this!"

I figured my days as a nursing student were probably over so I repeated my confession. "I gave her a good shaking."

The concerned looks from my peers helped me a bit but the teacher's incredulous look scared me speechless. I stood quietly waiting for whatever punishment was coming.

"I cannot believe you would do such a thing," she said hotly, "you know this could have very serious repercussions."

"My method may not have been by-the-book but it seems to have worked for Patty." I muttered. "She's bathed today and has been much more caring towards her daughter. In fact her whole behavior has improved."

My instructor shook her head at me. "Well we will have to wait and see won't we?"

Not to belabor the telling of this tale I will only add that after this unusual form of treatment Patty was discharged home within that same week. I got a severe reprimand from the teacher and the Director of the nursing school but was allowed to continue in the program.

I have often wondered how Patty made out, and if she ever remembers me giving her that shock. One thing is certain, I don't think I'll ever forget her.

Being in Control

Brian was over six feet tall. He was in his early forties and had been in the chronic care hospital for nearly five years, with a muscle wasting disease. This had debilitated him to the point that he needed total nursing care.

The first time that I met him, he struck me as being a very private person. He would never initiate a conversation, and seldom seemed to want to chat, hard as I tried to get him to talk. So most of the time I worked with him in silence.

However, I always liked to know something about my patient's background so I continued to try to get him to open up and speak.

"So Brian, " I said, as I rolled him towards me so I could wash his back. " Where were you born?"

"I know you were not born here, " he said. "Your accent gives you away.'

"That's right. I was born and raised in England. But, never mind me, what about you." I smiled. "Tell me something about yourself, that's if you want to."

"I was born here, " he said.

"Here? I said. You mean in Canada?"

His large, blue eyes twinkled. "Well, where do you think I meant?" I grinned and shook my head. "Okay, that was a dumb question. So you're a Canadian. But, that still doesn't disclose much else about you."

He gave me a sly look. "Let's just say, I was born outside of the city, and that'll be enough for now. I don't like to divulge too many secrets all at once. If I did that we'd have nothing further to discuss when you see me another time."

"That's fine. Anyhow, Brian, I am sure we will have many more opportunities to uncover your past. We've at least made a start."

He hooted with laughter. "If you say so nurse. Far be it for me to disagree with you, especially when you've got me in this position." His morning bath completed I started to dress him.

Dressing a person who is unable to give any assistance is not the easiest of tasks. It requires a lot of rolling the patient from side to side while tugging and working to arrange their clothing so that there are no tucks or creases. Brian allowed me to put him through the many moves until he was ready to be transferred into his wheelchair.

"Okay," I said, in a jocular voice, as I placed a cover over his long legs." You wait here for me until I can come and get you up."

He glared at me. "And, just where the hell do you suppose I can go?" His frustration was evident in the tone of his voice, and this sudden change in him took me completely off guard.

Seeing the surprised look on my face, he pursed his lips. "Hey, I'm sorry for snapping at you like that. Still, would you believe it, nurse, if I told you that at one time I was a very good athlete. I know, you'd probably never think it looking at me now."

"Yes Brian, I do believe you." I touched his arm gently. And, I am sorry for what I said to you. It was very thoughtless of me."

"It's alright, nurse" His tone quieter. "I know you didn't mean any harm. But, have you any idea what it feels like to be trapped in a body that can't do anything like mine?"

"No Brian." I shook my head. "I have no idea of how it feels. I am sure though it cannot be an easy thing to live with. "You've got that right. In fact, it's a bit like being alive in a sense, yet also dead in another. At least that's the way it is for me sometlmes."

Standing at the side of his bed looking down on this man's once vibrant body, now paralyzed, I could see why he felt the way he did. His lower limbs were deformed and twisted, and his long fingers had taken on the shape of claws.

I struggled to find the right words to tell him that in spite of all this he was still very much a living, breathing, person.

He stared up at me with a quizzical expression. "So nurse, what are you so deep in thought about? Are you going to be telling me that I should just be glad that I am living? I hope not. I've already heard that too many times."

"No, Brian," I shook my head. "I'm not going to tell you anything like that. I would just say that although you are limited in your activities because of your disease, you can talk and you are able to communicate your feelings. Surely, that is important?" I looked at him. "What do you think?"

He raised his thick, dark eyebrows and frowned. "Yes! Yes, you are right, I can talk. But, what else can I damn well do? Will you tell me that, nurse?"

"Well, for starters," I grinned at him. "You can put an end to all this chitchat, and let me go and get the rest of my work done. If you don't then you'll be looking at one unemployed nurse."

His pleasant face broke into a broad grin. "Am I hearing you right? You are telling me that I do have some control after all. If I keep you in here too long gabbing you'll be out of a job."

"Yes, that's what I'm saying." I tapped him gently on the top of his head. "So you see, you do have some power. In fact, everyone has, to a certain degree. It's not always easy to understand how much or what it is, but it is a fact."

"I like that a lot." He laughed aloud. "Yes, that's good to know. Thanks, nurse."

"No problem, glad I could help."
I moved towards the door. "Anyway, Brian, I'm pleased we've had this time together to talk, and that you felt comfortable enough with me that you were able to vent some of your feelings. I just hope we can do it again." I waved to him. "Now, I really do have to get going. Okay?"

"Okay. Yes." he said. "Yes, I'll let you go." He winked. "Just, as long as you promise to come back soon to get me up in my chair."

As I walked out of his room, I could still hear him chuckling. From that initial meeting, Brain and I shared many enjoyable conversations. I discovered that below all his physical limitations, Brian had a wonderful zest for life, and a great sense of humor. I'm glad I had the chance to get to know him.

The Problem needed Padding

"Before we begin, I have to tell you nurse I don't walk very well."

My elderly patient smiled at me. Her bright blue eyes sparkled, lighting up her small, lined features. She watched me closely as I prepared everything to get her out of bed.

Mrs. Bailey had come to our ward because of breathing difficulties. She was on numerous medications and the plan was to get these reduced and her respiratory condition improved so that she could return home. I knew about these problems but no one had mentioned anything wrong with her feet.

"My family doctor tells me that it is all related to getting older, but I think there is something wrong with the soles of my feet."

Mrs. Bailey grabbed at my hand as I went to remove her bed covers. She grinned saucily. "Old age nurse, you know, isn't for weaklings or cowards."

I chuckled. "You've got that right," I said. " Even so, there's a lot of things that can be done to make life tolerable, when one is getting on in years."

"That sounds really lovely," she said. " But I don't think that there is anyway that you can help me to walk better."

I had Mrs. Bailey sitting on the edge of her bed ready to stand up. I could see she had a prominent dowager's hump, which seriously affected her posture. To properly assess her ambulatory status I needed to see how well she could stand. Helping her into the upright position was easy. Then I saw that she had all her weight balanced on the sides of her feet. There was obviously a problem with something. No one could walk properly like that.

"This really isn't very comfortable nurse, " My patient said grimacing. " I would like to sit down again please. If you don't mind?"

"You certainly don't stand very well," I said, letting her back down. "I'd like to take a good look at those feet of yours, if that's fine with you?" She laughed. "I can tell you now that they are a real sorry sight"

Mrs. Bailey was accurate in her description. They were an awful mess to see. Because she had been trying to walk on the sides of her feet, there were huge calluses on both outer edges. On closer inspection of the areas under her toes, I saw that she had hardly any normal padding left. When I touched this part of her foot, she winced.

"Ouch!" she said. "That hurts."

"I'm not surprised, " I told her. "The problem is that you have almost lost all of the fatty tissue that protects the heads of the metatarsal bones. Your doctor was correct in one way because it often happens when we age. I can, however, do something that will ease it."

She squeezed my hand. "If you can help me so I can get around in less pain I'll be eternally grateful."

"Well, it just so happens," I smiled. " You have a nurse who has been helping people for many years with all sorts of foot problems." I gently touched the soles of her feet. "These won't be at all difficult to fix."

Mrs. Bailey clapped her hands and smiled broadly. "Aren't I the lucky one getting you today."

"I don't know about that." I said. "I'm just pleased that I know I can help you."

I moved towards the door of her room. "I'll have to go and get a few things but I'll be right back."

Mrs. Bailey intently watched me as I worked. "What are you doing that for?" she asked, as I applied pads to the undersides of both feet.

"Well, as I said, you've lost most the protective covering for these bones." I gently touched the area in question. "What we need to do is give you something that will work much the same way. This padding will do that."

I was often asked to provide foot care to patients, so I always kept a good supply of dressing material in my locker. In no time at all I had the calluses on her feet filed down, and the pads in place.

"Now, before you're discharged," I said, putting my equipment away. "I'll make you a couple of them, which you can take home and remove when you get into bed at night."

I helped Mrs. Bailey up again so she was standing by the side of her bed. "How do your feet feel now?"

She beamed. "They do feel a bit strange, but at least they don't hurt as much."

"Here, let me help you try and walk on them." I took a firm hold of her arm.

We started very slowly. Mrs. Bailey gingerly taking small steps. "I'm walking just like an infant getting around for the first time." She chortled loudly.

I laughed with her. "You'll soon get the hang of it again. The sides of your feet were never meant to be used like soles."

In a short time, she did that. What was more satisfying to see was the change in her attitude. She smiled more and talked excitedly about the different things she was going to be able to do once discharged.

On the day she was due to go home Mrs. Bailey came down to the desk on the arm of a friend. Her gentle face held a broad grin as she again thanked me. Before she left the ward, we embraced. In my mind's eye I can still see her waving back to me as she walked slowly away from the nurse's station.

His Other Talent

Boredom can be debilitating at times. On a hospital ward, it sometimes is the difference between a slow or a swift recovery. One of our regulars on the cardiac-respiratory unit knew how to beat the odds on this ever happening to him.

Dave a tall, rotund, elderly man with irregular heart beat and chronic emphysema was in to have his medication regimen checked. Although he was not able to do too much, he still made it part of his regular routine to visit any patients who were confined to their beds.

I knew that Dave had emigrated from Ireland many years earlier. I often thought that he must have kissed the blarney stone before coming to Canada. He loved to joke around and enjoyed seeing people laugh.

I remember on one admission he carefully filled the urine specimen bottle with flat ginger ale. The color is similar and in the rush to pick up the samples, no one spotted the difference.

After trying to analyze it, the lab sent us sarcastic note. "This patient has a real problem. His urine is made up entirely of a flat carbonated beverage."

They made several irate suggestions about what we should be doing before sending them any more samples. Dave got a scolding from some of the staff, but because his prank did give us a good chuckle, we let him off lightly.

This genial man liked to give assistance us in any way he could. We usually had someone on the floor that wasn't doing so well and Dave would go in and try to cheer that person up.

Although I remember Dave for the way, he tried to keep everyone's spirits in high gear it is his other talent, which became known. We discovered that he also had the ability to carry a tune.

100

Over the course of several days, everyone had heard this one tune played nearly every hour on the radio. It was as if the disc jockeys could not help themselves; they had to play it. After a while most of the staff groaned whenever they heard it. Alternatively, they found themselves humming along with the musical rendition.

Jane and I had our patients settled for the night and we were back at the nurse's station. I was getting charts ready while she was working on the doctor's orders. Suddenly someone coming down the north hallway singing at the top of their voice shattered the peacefulness of the ward.

"What the heck is that all about?" I looked with amazement at Jane.

She shrugged her shoulders, "I don't know, but we'd better go and see who is making all that ruckus. If he wakes the others up we'll have a mutiny on our hands."

We both moved out from behind the desk and stood together at the top of the hallway. The sight that met our eyes caused us both to start laughing.

Dave was coming towards us, dressed only in a short, blue, hospital gown, which barely covered his knees. He was swinging his cane as he walked and his deep voice loudly sang, "Oh! Lord it's so hard to be humble, when you're perfect in every way."

It was obvious that Dave's ears had been assailed once too often with this popular ditty. He had been unable to stop himself. Hearing it repeatedly on the air, this genial outgoing man had been compelled into singing it aloud.

As he came towards us, he gave a saucy wink. "Well what do you think girls, will I make it to stardom?"

Grinning at him I said, "Well I don't know about you becoming a star, but if you've roused too many patients from their slumber you'd better run and hide."

"That's for sure, " Jane told him.

"Now come on you two." Dave said. "Some folk enjoy being serenaded."

My co-worker turned to me. "I'm going to leave you to get this fellow back to his bed."

Dave looped his arm through mine. "Guess you've got the task of returning me safely to my room. I couldn't help myself you know. That tune has been buzzing around in my head. "

"I know, it's done the same to all of us. "I gently squeezed his arm. "You're a pip you know that."

"Well, someone has to keep everyone's spirits up around here. I like to think I help do that."

"You do that alright. It's a treat having you on the ward. You have a marvelous way with people and that's a real gift."

As we walked into his room, his roommate greeted him. "I told you you'd be brought back to your room by one of the nurses. I should have taken you up on your bet which one it'd be."

Amid much laughter and gentle ribbing from both of these elderly men, I finally got this patient settled back in his bed.

As I switched off their light, I heard Dave softly sing the tune again. "Oh! Lord it's so hard to be humble when you're perfect in every way.

I thought, he really does have a fine voice as well as all his other attributes. "Shush now. " I said. "It's time you both got some sleep."

We only had a couple of patients who had heard the noise and they were soon resettled. As For Dave, we never heard him sing that tune aloud again. His one performance had served its purpose.

Money Doesn't Always Count

"I will give you whatever you want Doc, " Mr. Currey said. "Just tell me that you can cure me, that's all."

"That's all Mr. Currey?" the specialist said. "That's quite a tall order."

This gentleman was a tobacco farmer. He had been on our unit many times before, over the last few years, for various health problems. He was a friendly, soft-spoken man and was an easy person to look after. He would quietly ask for help. He never demanded anything, which made his present request seem even more odd.

I was in his room at the same time that the medical team was doing their rounds. The doctors stood in a group at the end of Mr. Currey's bed. They took turns looking at his chart and the requisitions of his tests.

The chief specialist kept conversing with the young interns, and med. students. My patient sat up stiffly in his bed; biting his nails, and anxiously watching all that was going on.

Mr. Currey suddenly started to have a coughing spasm. One of the doctors motioned to me to give my patient some assistance.

The tissue that I gave him was soon flecked with blood. I opened it up so the team was also able to see it.

"What's the matter with me doc? "Mr. Currey quietly muttered. "Bet it's nothing that you can't fix."

The doctor shook his head. "I wouldn't bet on anything at the moment if I was you sir. Your lungs are not looking good at all."

The old gentleman laughed. "Well this here, nurse, says you're one of the best doctors around, "he chuckled. "So I am not worried one bit. I know you'll get me all sorted out."

I felt my face flush with embarrassment over this man's remarks. I wanted to run out of the room and hide. Instead I stood silent, and just shrugged my shoulders and nodded at the doctor.

The specialist grinned at me. "Well, it's certainly always nice to know someone on the staff here thinks I'm good at what I do."

He turned back to Mr. Currey. "But in your case, there's not really a lot I can offer you."

My patient shook his head. "You're joshing me doc, isn't that right nurse?" He peered intently at me.

Having read the results of the numerous tests this man had been given I knew that his diagnosis was guarded. I couldn't answer him. I just looked back at him and tried to convey that I cared about how he was feeling right then.

"I'm a wealthy man you know, doctor, " Mr. Currey said. "I've worked hard all of my life and I've been careful with my money."

The specialist smiled. "I'm pleased to hear that, but that's not going to be of much help to you now. It isn't your worth that's in doubt it's your health."

The medical team was starting to move towards the door. "Just a minute doctors, " Mr. Currey loudly ordered. "As I told you earlier I'll give you whatever it takes, money or anything, as long as you can guarantee to make me better."

"I wish it was that easy." The chief doctor said. He looked concerned as he added. "As soon as we've decided on some sort of treatment, we'll get right back to you."

My patient looked devastated. His large round face turned red, and he bit his bottom lip. "Is that all you can damn well do for me?" he yelled at them. "What the hell good is my money if it won't give me what I want."

No one on the team gave him an answer, so he turned to me and bellowed; "My money was always suppose to provide me with anything I wanted. What good is it if it can't? I might just as well be a pauper."

I was not sure how to respond to this outburst. I could see and feel his intense anger over what he'd been told.

He glared at me. "You lied to me. You told me they'd be able to help me."

Mr. Currey," I said softly, "I'm sorry that you're feeling this way, but it is a natural human response. It's okay to be angry." Still, I think it is important for you to remember that the medical team will do everything they can possible do. That's their job and they are good at it."

"Damn, " he said. "That's not good enough."

"Look, maybe it would be better if you wait till the doctors have a plan of care. Then you'll know exactly what can be done for you."

I gently touched his callused, hard surfaced hands that lay clenched on the top covers. I peered intently into his wrinkled, tired drawn face.

"How does that sound?"

He gave a deep heartfelt sigh, and burrowed down under the bed-covers. "I've got to think about it, " he muttered. "And, look I'm sorry I yelled at you."

"That's alright." I nodded. "I know all of this must been difficult, and you just needed to vent your feelings."

This elderly gentleman learned later that he had lung cancer, and his only course of treatment was radiation. He chose not to take any of it, but instead sorrowing went back home to his farm.

I learnt from this mans experience, that people sometimes consider as true that their money can buy them anything. Moreover, it is often only when a person becomes ill or infirm that the real value of their health is recognized.

A Negative Reaction

Mrs. Grier refuses to allow me to provide her with any care. As I wrote these words in the lady's chart, I experienced many mingled emotions. In all the years that I'd been, practicing nursing I'd never had a patient turn down my care. It gave me an odd feeling. Nevertheless, I thought that my approach with this lady had been the proper one and I had behaved appropriately given the circumstances.

These events all occurred on a medical unit one evening while I was on the night shift. There was an unwritten rule on that ward, that if a patient's status warranted it then their family could stay with them overnight. This had been the crux of the dispute I had had with this lady.

Mrs. Grier's roommate was very ill, and it was decided that this patient's husband could stay with her. Arrangements were made to provide him with a recliner chair so he could try and get some rest.

Entering the semi-private room that they shared, I moved across to speak with Mrs. Grier. Mrs. Peters, the other occupant, was blocked from view by the heavy curtains that surrounded her bed.

"Hello! " I said cheerfully." How are you feeling this evening Mrs. Grier?"

"I'm not at all well, " she snapped back at me, " and having that man, " she angrily pointed to the drapes, " hiding behind there makes me feel much worse."

"Why do you say that?" I asked her. "You can't see him." She stared angrily at me. " I can hear him breathing so I know he's in there."

I could not believe this lady's demeanor towards a fellow patient. Striving to keep my voice under control, I said, " I don't understand why you're so upset that Mrs. Peters husband has permission to stay with her."

"Oh! You don't understand, " she said sarcastically. " Well let me tell you why I'm upset. I'm a sick woman too, " she screamed, "and none of you seem to care."

"Please, " I said. "There is no need to yell like that. As you can see I'm right here beside you."

"I'll yell, she said, " as much as I want to until you get rid of that man."

"I can't do that. Your roommate really needs her husband to be with her this evening."

"She's damn well no sicker than I am, " Mrs. Grier hollered. " Why should she get all this preferential treatment?"

It was difficult for me but keeping my voice calm, I bent down close to Mrs. Grier. "If you were not ill, " I said, " you wouldn't be here in hospital. But your room mate requires a little more attention than we can give her right now, and her husband has offered to help us out."

"What's the matter with her anyway?" she said tersely. " I know her sort just putting on a command performance to get all this extra attention."

At that point, I saw Mr. Peters had come out from his wife's bedside. He motioned that he wanted to speak to me.

"You see there he is, just as I told you, " Mrs. Grier said smugly.

Mr. Peters told me he would leave his wife's room. He did not want to be the cause of any distress for the other patient in the room. I assured him that there was no way that he had to do this, and that if need be we'd move Mrs. Grier some place else.

It was when I suggested that she move to another room that Mrs. Grier accused me of being uncaring. She shoved me away from her bedside. Her face flushed and she screamed. "Don't you ever come anywhere near me again. And, I intend to let you're supervisor know how badly you've treated me."

When I came on duty the next night and learned that Mrs. Peters had passed away. I felt that my actions the previous shift had been justified.

In spite of that, Mrs. Grier refused to allow me anywhere near her. She never offered one word of regret about the fact that her roommate had died. That hurt me more than her attack on my nursing.

The Special Surprise

Mrs. Taylor was a middle-aged lady who had come to the ward because of her heart problems. She was a lady who loved life and was very active in the community. To her this visit to the hospital was nothing but a minor irritation and she would soon be out-and-about back to her old routine.

That did not turn out to be the case although we all would have loved to be able to support her positive attitude. The reason, however, why she remains so firmly in my store of memories is because of what she did for her granddaughter.

"How are you today?" I greeted her as I entered her room. "I'm just fine thank-you Nurse. How are you?"

I smiled at her. "I'm well thank-you but I'm supposed to be the one who asks you that, not the other way around!"

Mrs. Taylor nodded her tousled grey head and chuckled. "Do you happen to know what those doctors have got planned for me today? I've been prodded and poked so much there ain't much left of me to look at."

She laughed aloud. I joined in with her.

"Actually today there is nothing scheduled that I know of. Why do you ask?"

"Because I'd like you to do something for me, if you will?" Brown eyes anxiously peered at me. I wondered what she was going to ask me to do.

Teasingly I said, "Well as long as it's nothing illegal there shouldn't be a problem."

"Oh! No. No No! It's nothing like that nurse. I just want you to help me with a surprise for my young granddaughter."

"That doesn't sound too bad, " I said, as I set her up for her morning care. "As soon as I've seen the rest of my patients

I'll be back and we can talk some more about this. How does that sound?"

Smiling she nodded. "Sounds fine to me."

Back at the desk, I spoke with my supervisor. "Mrs. Taylor has asked me to help her do something she's planning for her granddaughter."

She pouted and looked stern. "Well as long as you feel you have enough time and you don't neglect your other patients. There is always the risk when you are doing personal business for a patient that you are going beyond the boundaries of being a caregiver. You need to use caution."

"I assure you I'll be most careful." I said.

"I hope you will." She said, as she resumed doing her paperwork.

The morning was flying past and I had not been back yet to see this lady. Finally, I had a few minutes to spare and I quickly walked down the hall towards her room.

Mrs.Taylor was sitting in her chair napping. Hearing me enter she roused and chuckled, "You've caught me snoozing again. I can't seem to keep my eyes open for very long anymore. Still never mind that for now. If you'll just come over and sit here I will explain what I need you to do, " she motioned for me to sit on her bedside.

"Okay." I said. So tell me what you're planning."

"Well, I have only one granddaughter as you know. That's her in that picture on my side-table." She pointed to the small gilt frame sitting amongst her possessions.

"She is a lovely young woman and has been so good to me, " her voice trembled. Taking a deep breath she added, " I just thought it would be a marvelous idea if I could give her a special gift. I'd like to do this while I'm still living so I could share some of her excitement and pleasure." She was watching me for a reaction.

"Do you think I'm being a silly old woman wanting to do something as that?" She rubbed at the tears that had come to her eyes.

"I've always believed nurse that it's best to give to those you love while you're with them, than leave them lots of things in a will. Anyway, when people do that it so often causes conflict amongst family members. That's another reason why I don't like it."

I patted her hand. "I think that's a lovely thought, and it certainly has a great deal of merit." I smiled.

"So what are you thinking of getting your granddaughter?"

"I would like her to have her very own car, " she said. "And so, that's what I'd want to give her."

My face must have mirrored surprise because Mrs. Taylor added. "You think that's too much?"

I shook my head. "No no! I think that would be a lovely gift. I'm sure she would be thrilled with it. But, do you have any kind of car in mind?"

"This is where I need your backing; I don't know very much about cars."

"Whoa! You're looking at the wrong person." I shrugged my shoulders. "I don't know much about them either."

"That doesn't matter." She grinned. "I've got it all worked out, so I'm sure that you can help."

I laughed aloud. "This should be interesting."

"What I need you to do is call around to some of the local car dealerships and see if they will send someone up to see me?" She gave me a slip of paper with these instructions on it. "Do you think that will be possible?"

"I don't see why not." I said. "But, I'd like to have some idea of how much you want to spend before I make any calls."

"Well I know a car doesn't come cheap." Mrs.Taylor smiled. "It'll likely cost a few thousand dollars and that's just fine. I'm not looking for a brand new car just a good secondhand one."

My patient's eyes started to flicker and I could see from her rapid breathing she was becoming tired. Rising up I helped her to get back into bed.

"I think it's time you took a rest." I said. "You leave all of this with me and I'll see what I can arrange."

"Yes, I have to admit I'm feeling a bit weary." She sighed deeply. "Thank-you so much for listening to me and for your offer to help."

As I made my way back to the nurse's station I wondered just how I was going to accomplish the task that this lady had set for me. I wasn't sure if a salesperson would come to a hospital even if they knew they were going to make a sale.

Later that day I decided it would be best to work on this project when I was at home. I told Mrs.Taylor my plan before leaving the ward and she agreed that was a good idea.

It turned out it was not as hard as I had anticipated, to get a salesperson to come and see this lady. When I explained what she wanted, I actually had a couple of dealerships who were willing to send someone in right away. I told them both I would get back to them as soon as I had spoken with this patient.

Mrs. Taylor greeted me warmly the next day when I entered her room. "Nice to see you again nurse."

"Well it's good to see you too, " I told her. "How are you?"

"Not as well as I'd like, but never mind that." She promptly sat up in her bed.

"Just come over here," she beckoned, "and tell me if you were able to get someone to sell me a car."

Standing by her bed I smiled, and nodded. "As a matter of fact I found two dealerships who were willing to send someone in to see you."

She clapped her hands and her small lined features lit up. "That's great. That's, wonderful."

I was delighted to make this lady happy. "We can talk about this later when you've decided which one you want to see."

"Lovely! Lovely! Lovely!" She clapped her hands again and smiled. I left her looking over the names of the two car dealerships.

Once I had completed, my morning work I went back in to see Mrs. Taylor. "So have you picked the one you want."

"Indeed I have, and I'd be most grateful if you would call him for me and make all the arrangements."

It was amazing how swiftly the dealer sent one of their sales people up to see this lady, and how quickly she was able to choose the type of car she wanted to buy. It seemed that it took no time at all before she had everything settled.

The day dawned when the car was to be delivered to her granddaughter's home address. Excitement from this lady was unmistakable. She could barely contain her feelings.

Before leaving the ward that morning, I went in to see her. "I'll be back on duty tonight." I said. "So I'll see you later."

"Oh! Nurse do you think my granddaughter will get her car today?" she looked uneasy as she voiced her concerns.

Standing beside her bed, I tried to reassure her. "I'm certain everything will be just fine and it will go just as you've planned."

"I couldn't have done it without your help." She grabbed hold of my hand.

Giving her hand a gentle squeeze, I placed the covers back around her. "I think you should just lie here and try to calm down until the day nurse comes on duty. And don't worry."

It seemed to take me ages to get to sleep when I finally got into bed. I kept thinking of Mrs.Taylor's granddaughter and the surprise she was going to get. She was lucky to have such a caring, loving grandmother.

Although my shift was not due to begin until eleven o'clock that night I chose to go in a bit earlier. Popping my head into Mrs.Taylor's room, I was surprised to see she was still awake.

Her face lit up with a big smile when she saw me. "What a day, what a day this has been nurse; I'm never going to forget it, it's been absolutely wonderful."

"So I take it everything went just as you hoped it would." I smiled back at her.

"Yes! Yes! Yes!" she gave a deep-contented sigh.

"My granddaughter got her car and they even remembered to put the big bow on the top of it, just as I asked them to do. I will have to call them and thank them. I'll do that later."

"Did your granddaughter come in to see you?"

"Oh yes and what a time we had. She scolded me of course, but in a nice way. It was grand seeing how happy she was with her gift." She sighed again. "I'm such a lucky lady to have been able to share this very special day with her."

"Well," I smiled at her, "I believe she is equally lucky to have a grandmother like you."

I was fixing her pillows and straightening her covers as we talked. "Now, " I said. "I'd better go and get started with my work, while you should try and get to sleep"

As I switched off the light, she bade me a weary sounding but happy, "Goodnight nurse."

Softly I replied, "Goodnight Mrs. Taylor, and pleasant dreams."

Not the Reaction I'd Hoped

"You're going to have to feed Mrs. Mills today, " the charge nurse ordered. " So you'd better allow yourself plenty of time. She can be rather difficult."

I had heard some of the other staff members grumbling about how long it took completing her care. As I had never been assigned to look after her I did not know why this was a problem. However, it was not long before I found out.

Entering her semi-private room, the first thing that I noticed was a large doll lying beside her in bed. It was a practice in this chronic care facility to give some of the older female patients' toys to hold and cuddle.

I gently touched Mrs. Mills on her shoulder, and made a movement to remove the doll. A small angry face with a pair of bright, beady, blue eyes glared at me, and one wrinkled, wiry hand tightly clutched the manikin to her chest.

"Hello." I said. "I'm your nurse today. Now, may I put this over on the side table for you?" I tried gently to pry the doll out of her hand.

There was no doubt in my mind that Mrs. Mills was not going to cooperate. The fixed expression of her narrow chin and the piercing look in her eyes spoke volumes. I decided it was probably best not to upset her.

I patted the hand that was gripping the figure. "It's alright, it can stay in bed with you, if that's what you want. I'll just get you set up so I can get you bathed before your meal-tray comes."

Ideally, I tried to give my patients their full morning bath before feeding them. But, on this particular day, my workload was extra heavy so I chose to just give Mrs. Mills a quick wash of her hands and face. She let me complete this procedure without any fuss, but when I tried to put her, teeth in she wouldn't open her mouth. She had her lips clamped like a vice.

"Now come on." I pleaded. "You need to have your dentures in so you can eat your food properly." Again I tried to gently open the small jaw, but it was clear from her scowl that she was not going to comply.

"Okay! Perhaps once your meal is here you'll feel differently." I replaced the teeth in her denture cup.

"I'll be back as soon as the meals are delivered." I moved towards the door.

Mrs. Mills was unable to do anything for herself as well as being aphasic, unable to answer or speak. I had an uncanny feeling, however, that she understood me, from the way her eyes watched my every move.

In this particular hospital, we always had one, or more, patients each day that needed to be fed. This could be a time-consuming task especially if there was a secondary problem with that individual.

We had several candy stripers, young teen volunteers, who assisted us with this. Nevertheless, none were allowed to feed Mrs. Mills. She was the hospital staff's sole responsibility.

The trays had all been delivered, and I decided to go and feed this lady. "Okay Mrs. Mills, " I said." Lets see what you've got for breakfast today." I moved the tray closer to her on her over-bed table.

She made no movement to grab at it, which many our patients often tried to do. I considered that was a good sign, and everything was going to be all right.

She watched me closely as I uncovered the containers of food. "But, first you do need to get your teeth in." I held her dentures ready and placed my hand under her chin waiting for her to open her mouth. .

It was obviously useless. Her mouth remained sealed. "That's fine by me. You do not want them so we will not bother with them." I positioned a terry-towel bib in front of her.

Her meal consisted of all soft food. She had cream of wheat, a soft poached egg and one slice of crustless, buttered toast.

"Okay, let's begin with your cereal," I said. I put the spoon in front of her mouth. It was amazing how quickly she opened her mouth and gulped the food in. I could hardly believe my good fortune. Especially, after all the fuss my peers had made about how difficult it was getting her to eat. Every time I positioned the spoon in front of her, she grabbed onto it. This, I thought is going to be a breeze.

After Mrs. Mills had eaten her first course, I looked closely at her face. For some strange reason, her cheeks were swelling out. I couldn't understand what was making them do that.

Then I realized that although Mrs. Mills was keen to get the food into her mouth she was not swallowing it. She had it all stored in her cheeks. Now what was I going to do?

"Please, Mrs. Mills," I begged." Swallow that food. I can't give you anything else, until you do, on account of you'll end up choking yourself."

This patient's rigid expression told me she was not going to do as I'd asked.

"Now look here, "I said crossly. " I really don't have time to spend trying to get you to eat properly. If you won't swallow I'm going to leave your meal here, and go and get on with my other work."

Two bright eyes glared into mine. Her cheeks, now looking like balloons, were chock-full of food.

I wonder I thought, if I placed a finger under her nose if that would help. This is how one can sometimes get a small child to take medicine.

Placing my index finger under my patient's nose did not get the response I had wanted. Instead, Mrs. Mills pursed her lips and ejected a steady stream of cream of wheat. It went all over my face and the front of my uniform.

"Oh! Yuck!" I yelled. I was taken aback by this turn of events. "Now look at what you've done. Why did you do that?"

Mrs. Mill's expression had not really altered, yet I could have sworn her eyes shone more brightly.

"Well, I hope you're satisfied." I was exasperated, but tried hard not to show this in the tone of my voice.

"I'll have to go and get this mess cleaned up. I'll be back later to give you the rest of your meal."

As I emerged from this lady's room, I ran into my supervisor who was coming down the hall. She stopped in her tracks and grinned." I see that you've just had a run in with our special patient." She laughed. "You have to admit it, she has a funny way with her."

"I don't know about being funny, "I muttered, "but she's definitely a difficult patient to feed. And, why does she keep all her food like that in her cheeks?"

"We don't really know, but we call her our little chipmunk. She does eat properly at times, but as you've obviously found out, she has a will of her own. Anyhow, you go and get yourself fixed up while I'll see if I can get her to take the rest of her breakfast."

There were many more occasions when I had this lady as part of my assignment. She was always the same. However, I never again tried the trick of putting my finger under her nose.

I learnt something from Mrs. Mills, never under-estimate a person's capability. Even when somebody may look as though they have no means to retaliate, they will find their own way of doing so!

Her Hidden Strength

"Hello." Pat's small, oval face looked tired as she greeted us. "I'm back again." She smiled. "But this will only be a short stay."

Emily, our daughter, is getting married in a week's time and I've got to be there." She turned her blonde head and gazed for a moment up at her husband. He touched her and nodded his head.

Mrs. Baker, or Pat as we all called her, had a rare form of cancer. She had come to the medical floor several months earlier for tests and exploratory work. It was then that she had learned of her diagnosis. She knew that it was a fast growing type, and that she didn't have much time left. Nevertheless, we all knew that she was determined to see her daughter get married.

Pat was in for her regular chemotherapy treatment. She arrived on the ward in a wheel chair, because of her weakened condition.

"If you just go down to your room, " I said, " I'll be along soon to see you."

As they headed down the hall, I felt a great sorrow for this lady. Pat had been married to Bill for twenty-four years with a son and a daughter. They had been planning their daughter's wedding for nearly a year and I knew how important this event was to both of them.

Entering her room to get Pat's paper work completed I found her already in bed. "Well love, " Bill leaned over and kissed his wife, "I can leave you now in this nurse's care. I'll be back tomorrow." He waved as he left the room.

"Oh! " Pat lay back against the pillow. "I feel so tired." She gave a deep sigh. "More than I've ever felt before, which worries me a bit, because I've just got to be alright for next week."

I looked anxiously at this woman's pale face, and deep set brown eyes. I wanted to be able to reassure her, that she would be with her daughter on her special day, but I couldn't because I really didn't know for sure if it was the truth.

After getting everything I needed completed, and her resettled, I left her to have a rest. The nurse's station, never a quiet place on admitting days, resembled a beehive of activity. The constant coming and going of staff as they got their patients admitted, kept everyone busy. Still, several of my peers who knew Pat well came over to me and inquired about her condition.

Shrugging my shoulders I said, "I really don't know, but once her Doctor has examined her we could ask him."

The young intern who had seen Pat was sitting at the desk. "Excuse me," I said. "How did you find Mrs. Baker?"

His expression was grim which immediately gave me an uneasy feeling. "How well do you know her?" He asked me.

"I've known her ever since she first came to this floor. Why?" I asked.

"Then you know that her prognosis is poor." He glanced through her chart. "Also she has lost a lot of weight, and this doesn't help."

"You know, " I said. "She wants to attend her daughter's wedding, which is in ten days. She's been planning this for a very long time." I looked intently at him. "She is going to be able to go to that, isn't she?"

"Yes, Mrs. Baker, told me all about that." He frowned. "Let's just say at the moment we're unsure of whether or not she'll be well enough to attend"

Pat started her chemotherapy treatments the following day. When undergoing this form of treatment she suffered greatly from nausea and vomiting. We never liked to see any of our patients going through this distress.

Her case history had been the one for discussion at conference time. It was well known that this patient wanted to

120

attend her daughter's wedding, and it was agreed we would do everything possible to help her. A special plan of care was drawn up, which would be shown to the patient for her approval before being put into action.

"You want me to stay in my bed most of the day, " she muttered, as she looked over the paper.

I smiled, "Yes. We all think that if you conserve your energy, and let us assist you with most of your daily activities, you'll get stronger."

At first Pat had been emphatic in her protests that she could manage most everything on her own. She soon, however, agreed that she did feel better with all the extra rest.

She frequently told us, "You're all spoiling me so much, I won't know how to manage when I go home."

The day before her daughter's wedding Pat had arranged to have a hairdresser come in and fix up her hair. It was quite sparse and fine and usually we would have done it for her but she wanted it to look extra special for the morrow.

"When will you be getting your hair done?" I asked her as I bathed her that day.

"She's coming in at one o'clock. Is that a bad time?"

"No. That should work out just fine." I said. "I'll see if I can get the special neck support so she can wash your hair while you're lying on a stretcher."

"Oh! My, "Pat gave a little laugh. "You are making me lazy."

"You lazy? Never!" I gently touched her cheek. "We're doing all this so you've got lots of pep for tomorrow."

Finally, the day of the wedding dawned. Everyone on the floor from the staff to the other patients was all caught up in the thrill of the occasion. Pat was sitting up in a wheelchair at the desk when we arrived for the day shift. Her small face, although pale, glowed with happiness.

"I've got everything ready." She said. "All I need is someone to help me get washed and dressed."

"Is that so? " I said. "Well, as soon as we our get report over with we'll be right in me-lady." Several co-workers and I gave her a little bow, which made her giggle.

"Thank-you, thank-you, thank-you all of you." Her voice wavered and shook. "I know that I couldn't have done it on my own."

"Okay!" I gently scolded. "That's enough of that. We do not want you getting all mushy on us. You need to save that for the wedding." I turned her chair around. "Let's put you back in your room for now."

We still had other patients to provide with care, but that morning everything seemed to go smoothly and we soon had our work done. The entire ward was waiting to see Pat emerge from her room in all her finery.

Her lilac silk dress was a perfect fit and she had shoes that matched. As she was wheeled out into the hall the ooh's and aah's that greeted her appearance caused her to start to cry.

Bill leant over and kissed her. He tenderly dried her tears. "Now, now let's not be having any of that already." He grinned at all of us. "She'll probably weep a bucket when she sees Emily coming down the aisle." He waved to us as they made their way of the ward.

It was an anti-climax for the rest of the shift. The day flew past and it was almost time for Pat to return to the floor. Bill brought her in followed by the wedding party, which brought the other patients out of their rooms to cheer. We all admired their gowns, and congratulated the happy couple.

When she was being put to bed that night Pat said, "This has been one of the most wonderful days of my life. Again, I can't thank you all enough for what you've done."

"You were the one who really did it." I playfully scolded. "You were the one who had the willpower and the strong faith; all we did was give you a little bit of a push."

"You are all very kind, " she said smiling happily. Then she closed her eyes.

Pat lived long enough to see the photographs and share them with us. Soon after that, she was gone.

What I learned from her was that nothing is impossible, if you put your whole mind to it, and believe you can. These attributes can overcome almost any obstacle.

A Patient's Influence

"Well, Mr. Digby, here you are again." I smiled at the large elderly man being wheeled onto the ward.

"Yup, " he said with a loud laugh. "I just love coming back to see all of you beautiful people. And, to get some more of that tender-loving-care."

"I don't know if we've got any of that in stock today." I said.

He grinned. "Now, nurse. I know that you folks here have lots of TLC to spare."

Mr. Digby had been a patient on our respiratory floor many times. He suffered from a chronic obstructive lung disease and needed to be on continuous oxygen. This tall, rotund man seldom grumbled about anything, although he suffered greatly with his disability.

Gathering up all of my equipment, I followed this couple down the hall. "You're going back into your usual room, " I said jokingly. "We've been keeping it just for you."

"Well......" he clenched his lips and breathed deeply through the nasal prongs attached to his oxygen tank. Forcefully he blew the air out. "To be honest with you, even though all you folks always take good care of me, I'd much rather not be coming back in again."

Patting him on his arm as I helped to transfer to the bed I said, " I know that, Mr. Digby. Let's just hope that your stay this time isn't long."

The reason for him coming in was to change his medication regime, and to assess whether he needed to go into a long-term facility. His wife worked outside of their home, and he really needed to have someone with him at all times.

I looked down at his anxious face, and saw that the tip of his nose and his lips were bluish in color. "It looks as if you need some extra help there." I said. "You're having a real hard time with your breathing."

"Suppose I go and see if the Doctor will order you an immediate ventolin treatment, and then I'll call down for it. You need to be comfortable before I start this." I laid the chart on his side table.

"Okey......Dokey, " he said, giving me a thumbs up signal.

Mrs. Digby had been sitting by the window absorbed in a magazine while I had been talking to her husband. She rose and came towards me.

"I've got to go now, as well, nurse or I'll be late for work. If there are any problems, you have the number where I can be reached."

Before leaving she went over and gave her husband a quick peck on the cheek. "See you tomorrow, " she said.

With some difficulty, he again muttered. "Okey dokey."

I quickly made my way down to the desk to get help for this mans breathing difficulties. Once he received the medication inhalant, I knew that he would be in less distress.

I was fortunate during my time working as a nurse to have the support of some exceptional physicians. Although I hadn't completed my basic training as a Registered Nurse, I was nearly always accepted as being a proficient care provider.

Being a Registered Nursing Assistant did not hamper my relationship with the doctors who were attending to any of my patients. Seeing Mr. Digby's doctor sitting in the nurse's station, I gave him a quick report of my patient's status and a ventolin treatment was duly ordered for him. These treatments were commonplace on this ward and usually gave the person having difficulty breathing instant relief.

When I returned to my patient's room, I was pleased to see he was much more comfortable, and he was sitting up in his bed reading the newspaper. "How are you feeling now?" I asked.

"Much, much better, " he answered giving me a broad grin. "Now, if I could just stay this way all day....but I suppose that's too much to hope for."

"Yes, " I nodded, " unfortunately that's something that you'll never be able to enjoy all the time anymore. Still, our goal is to find a way that will improve your level of breathing so you can be more active."

Giving me another smile, he said, "Sounds dandy to me."

"Perhaps later on we can talk about some of the things you'd like to be able to do." I said.

"Okey, dokey." He replied.

I touched him lightly on his arm. "I've got to leave you for a little while longer, but if you need me for anything just use your call bell."

"Okey dokey, " was once again his cheery answer.

In fact that's the very reason why this man is locked in my memory because of the way he would say, "okey dokey, " when asked how he was doing or how his day was going. It was his favorite reply and he constantly used it.

This phrase was picked up and spoken by almost everyone who happened to meet him. It was frequently heard at the desk and was the cause for some good-natured ribbing. When the person let it slip, we all knew right away that they had been in to see this jovial man.

It was as if we could not help ourselves, he had had such an Influence on us. However, I recall those two little words often brightened many of an otherwise stressful day on that ward. Consequently, no one really minded that he had got us all to say them.

I would like to be able to tell you that Mr. Digby or Mr. Okey Dokey as we affectionately ended up calling him improved enough that he was able to go home, but I cannot. His chronic obstructive lung disease ultimately was too much for him. He slipped away one night, never waking from a deep sleep. I hope, somehow, he knew/knows that his cheery personality gave us much pleasant relief.

A Disagreement of Sorts

Mrs. Franks roared with laughter when I asked her husband. " Have you ever had surgery?"

She was making such a noise that for a brief minute I feared she might have been going into a fit. I peered at her with concern until she calmed down.

This was a standard question, and one I had to ask every patient. I was not sure why this man's wife had reacted as she had but was soon to find out.

Mr. Franks paused for a moment before he angrily muttered, " I most certainly have."

Just as quickly his wife, said, "Oh, no you have not. That wasn't any surgery."

Her husband bristled with indignation, his square jaw stiffened and his face turned red. " Maybe it wasn't to you but I know what I went through, you don't."

Mrs. Franks laughed aloud again. " Honestly nurse have you ever heard anything so ridiculous. Men are such babies."

I shook my head, " That's not exactly true, " I said, " I've seen as many women go all to pieces after surgery as men."

"There you are, "Mr. Franks said smugly, "You women are just as much softies as you always say we are."

The atmosphere in the room was tense. Husband and wife glaring at each other, and I was caught in the middle. I thought it best to try to put a stop to this conversation before it got any worse.

Facing them both I said, "Look I don't know what the procedure was that you had Mr. Franks, but from what you're saying I gather to you it was major. So all I need to know from you sir, " I looked at Mr. Franks, "is what was it?"

Mrs. Franks smirked. "Yes Tom, why don't you tell the nurse exactly what surgery you underwent."

My patient sat on his bed and I could see he was fuming. He scowled at his wife.

"Alright, " I said, " let's leave that question and...go on....".

"Just stop it, will you. Stop it, " he yelled at his wife." He turned away from her and looked at me. "She can't leave it alone. She knows it annoys me."

I felt I was in over my head. This had never happened to me before. Obviously, my question to Mr. Franks had sparked off a response from him that had irked his wife. Well that was their problem not mine. They were the ones who were going to have to deal with it.

Once his wife had left, my patient relaxed and even gave me a warm smile. "I'm sorry you had to hear all that, nurse, but my wife and I have an ongoing difference of opinion about what happened to me."

"All I'm going to do is put a yes to that question about surgery. " I said. "You can go into more detail with the doctor when he or she comes in to do your physical."

Once I had collected all the information that I needed, and I was about to walk out of his room, Mr. Franks grabbed hold of my arm. "Don't you want to know what it was?"

I shook my head. " No it really doesn't matter. " I tried to remove his hand. "As I said, you can tell your doctor."

His hand was tightly, gripping my arm and I wanted it removed. "You're hurting me and I want you to let go."

"Oh! I'm sorry. I didn't mean anything by that. I'm sorry nurse. I am sorry. It's just I get so upset about this."

I stepped back rubbing my arm, " That's okay." I walked towards the door of his room. "I'll be in to see you later. Your doctor should be with you soon."

When I relayed what had happened, to a member of the medical team, the doctor gave a deep chuckle.

"I bet I know what he thinks was surgery." He smiled at me. Come on, can't you guess what it is nurse?"

"To tell the truth at the moment I don't care. All I know is that the behavior of that husband and wife while I was trying to collect that man's history wasn't fitting."

"Now nurse." The doctor scolded. "You know that patients get uptight about coming into hospital. That's probably all it was, a bad case of the jitters. Plus he seems, from what you've told me, to have an ongoing disagreement with his wife, over this."

Later I noticed the intern smiling and talking with the resident. He grinned when he saw me.

"I was right on about that patient of yours. His major procedure was a vasectomy. So you see nurse, it all depends on one's perception of what is surgery."

"I guess you're right. Did you tell Mr. Franks that's not considered to be surgery."

Giving a loud laugh he said, " No nurse I did not. I'm going to let you tell him."

For the record, I never did pluck up enough courage to inform him of this. I felt that he seemed to have marital problems enough without adding more fuel to the fire.

The Early Christmas

"Am I going to get to celebrate Christmas this year?" Tracy's thin, young, face looked tearful as she asked me this question. As it was only July and my patient was suffering from a chronic heart condition, that I knew was terminal, I didn't want to give her an immediate answer.

She had often told me how much she loved this special season and what it meant to her. Her definition was always the same. "It's the ultimate expression of God's love. And it's simply the best, best time of the year."

Tracy peered at me patiently waiting for a reply. I couldn't bring myself to tell her that she might not have enough time left, because I wasn't sure that was the truth. So what could I tell her?

I stood silent my thoughts jumbled, wondering what to say. Suddenly, like a bolt out of the blue I got a brilliant idea. Why not have early celebrations for her?

I smiled. "Tracy, I don't see why you can't hold Christmas. But how would you feel about having a special party just for you; an early one?"

Her eyes opened wide, making her delicate, pale features appear much smaller. "Wow! That sounds like a great idea, " she said." When can I have it nurse? When can I have it?"

I smiled at her enthusiasm. "Just as soon as it can all be arranged." I said. "It shouldn't take all that long to set things up."

When I spoke with some of my co-workers, they thought it was a lovely idea. Tracy's parents were eager also to help. They had been having a lot of difficulty seeing their only child suffering and not able to do very much for her. This would be an opportunity, they both said to do something practical. They knew that it would make their daughter happy, as well as give them satisfaction.

Once the word of our plans got around, we had offers of help from all quarters: nurses who wanted to make decorations or goodies, to doctors who wished to donate money.

It took a week to get everything in place. I arranged to have Tracy taken down to the Physiotherapy department, on the day we decided to hold the party. Her parents had fixed the decorations and the eats. The staff had bought and wrapped all the gifts.

The thrill on the ward was unmistakable as we scurried around getting her room ready. Some of the other patients wanted to join in the excitement. There were many helpful suggestions given.

As she was wheeled into her room, she let out a gasp, " Oh! Oh! It's all like Christmas." Tears streamed down Tracy's face. A lump formed in my throat. I heard a couple of nurse's cough as if clearing their own.

"Oh! Look, look," Tracy cried out. " I've even got a tree." She pointed to the small pot that sat on her bedside table. We had adorned the pine-tree with little, colored lights and Tracy's mother had placed a star on the top.

"Oh! And look Mum...Dad...I've got presents too." She clapped her hands.

Those of us in her room were unsure of what we should be doing. Emotions were running high, and our young patient was not the only one shedding a tear. Several of us sniffed as we rummaged in our pockets for Kleenexes.

Still I wanted to say something. " We...we.. are really pleased Tracy that you like all of this, and Happy Christmas."

"Like it I love it. Thank-you, thank-you all so much." Her eyes sparkled, and she beamed at all of us.

"Oh! Mum............Dad.. This is so perfect. Isn't it?" Her parents nodded

She glowed with delight as she looked around her room. Suddenly, she began to cry again and her mother gently took her in her arms. "It's alright my love, " she whispered. "This is

130

all just for you. We know how much Christmas means to you and we wanted to be able to celebrate it with you."

"That's right Kitten, " Tracy's Dad murmured.

"You've all been very kind." Her Dad smiled at us.

"We enjoyed doing it, " I said, looking at my peers." Didn't we?" They nodded in agreement.

Tracy and her mother had been looking at some of her gifts and had become emotional and teary again. That's when Tracy's dad lovingly placed his arms around them both and we all crept out of her room.

I wish I could tell you that Tracy enjoyed another Yuletide in December, but it was not to be. Nevertheless, for a little while that summer she had given us the marvelous opportunity to share with her in a lovely celebration of that season.

Out of Sight out of Mind

The isolation wing in the acute care hospital is also a hectic area. While attending school to get my Registered Nurse's diploma I was working as a relief nurse which meant that I worked on many different floors and that included this one.

Usually because of the type of patients and their major health problems, the nursing staff would be run off their feet doing numerous dressings and providing care. There could be surgical cases that had developed a bad wound infection or some who required to be isolated for their own safety. The problems were many and varied.

This particular period was even busier because of one lady whose needs were greater than anyone had ever before encountered. Her condition was extreme and created a lot of extra work for the staff on that unit.

I was welcomed warmly by the regular staff when I appeared on the ward. Although I wasn't allowed to administer medications or do the major dressing changes the warmth of their greeting told me they were pleased to see me.

"What we will have you do is look after the lighter cases, " the head nurse said. "That will be most helpful."

"And you can keep an eye out for any call-lights. This will give us the time we need to work in the rooms with those patients who require extra attention."

Each patient had a room of his or her own and every door was kept shut against possible cross contamination. Before one entered a room hands had to be thoroughly washed, and sterile gear had to be put on. Then before leaving, the same procedure was carried out. Once outside the patient's room the clothing and masks would be discarded.

Mrs. Woran was in that area because she had an enormous open area on her back. This was due in part to her poor health status but was also related to the fact that she had been allowed to lie in bed for months on end without anyone turning her. Consequently the skin on her back had broken open and she had a huge wound that had become infected. It was a disturbing sight. However, as this lady was also a paraplegic she had no feeling around that area. She had no idea of the extent of her skin breakdown.

One important facet of this lady's personality remains in my mind. Mrs. Woran was one of the most meticulous patients I'd ever met. She would insist on having a complete bed-bath every day, along with body oils and powders that she had brought with her. Her hairdresser would come in twice a week to do her hair and she had a manicurist do her nails.

She told me. "I like to always keep myself looking chic for my husband."

"I think that's a delightful thing to want to do. I smiled. But you know part of the reason you're now here is because of what you're husband didn't do?"

"I know the doctors have already gone over that. Mrs. Woran smiled. "I am a strong-willed woman, as you have probably gathered, the way I like my own way about things. My husband tried to get me off my back many times but I'd refuse to do it."

"So, what I hear you saying, I think, is it's partly your own fault."

She nodded, " Yes nurse. My husband has been very good to me. I'm sure that he doesn't like to see me in here anymore than I like being here."

"You do know, it is going to take quite a long time before you will be able to go home, " I said.

"Yes, I know that," Mrs. Woran sighed. "The doctors have told me that I have to get a skin graft once the infection has gone." I nodded, " That's quite right. They can't do anything to it until it's absolutely clean of all infection."

"They're planning on taking some skin from my thighs to fill in the hole, " she said.

She gave a little laugh. "I just hope that doesn't mean my legs will look all funny after they do that."

I was amazed. This lady was worrying about how her legs would look instead of thinking of the benefits it meant to her back. I smiled.

" Mrs. Woran, you will have a little scarring on your legs but it's something that has to be done if your wound is ever going to heal."

She again laughed. "You must be thinking I'm a very vain woman. I'm thinking only about the changes it will mean to my legs, and not how it is going to repair the hole in my back."

Actually, Mrs. Woran was right in a way I thought she had her priorities mixed up regarding her health needs. She spent several months on that unit so I frequently provided her with her basic care.

I always had the feeling that because Mrs. Woran could not see or feel the extent of her problem that she did not consider it to be of importance. It was out of sight so she kept it out of her mind. This still did not deter from my finding her an interesting lady.

A Call for Desperate Measures

The Registered Nurse and I entered the medical ward to begin the night shift. This was the seventh night on duty and we were looking forward to completing it, so we could get a couple of days off.

To our surprise, we saw that the head-nurse, Mrs. Brent was standing at the desk.

Sheila and I looked inquiringly at each other.

"What on earth is she doing here?" I whispered.

"Haven't a clue, " Sheila whispered.

As we came nearer to the desk, I saw that Mrs. Brent's face was a deep red and she glowered at us.

"Good evening Mrs. Brent, " we said in unison.

Speaking through gritted teeth Mrs. Brent said, " It is not a good evening. In fact I shouldn't even have to be here, but because of what you've both done I am."

Sheila tightly gripped my arm. "What is she talking about?" she softly said in my ear.

"There's no point in either of you trying to cover up your deed, " she snapped. "What did you forget to do this morning before you went off duty?"

Again, we both looked at each other trying to delve into one another's thoughts. Whatever was our head-nurse on about? My peer shrugged, and I raised my eyebrows in bewilderment. Neither of us had a clue what was wrong.

We had worked together often and had never been faced with a problem that we could not resolve. I shook my head hoping for some enlightenment.

"You needn't both stand there pretending that you don't know what I'm talking about, " Mrs. Brent snapped. She scowled. "This is serious business and I'm not one bit amused by your off-hand behavior."

"I'm sorry, " Sheila said quietly, " but neither of us can think what it is your referring to. What was it that we forgot?"

"What are the specific rules in this hospital regarding restraints?" she said crossly.

It was then that I had an awful feeling in my gut and I knew what we had not remembered. That had to be the reason why she was here.

"The rules are, "Sheila said, "that in extreme circumstances restraints can be used."

"That's correct, " Mrs. Brent said. "But what do you never, never, ever not do?"

Oh! Here it comes. I thought. Now we are in deep trouble. I knew instinctively what she was going to say.

"You left Mr. Bagsley trussed up as nothing I have ever seen before." she banged the top of the desk.

"The poor man couldn't move a muscle." She wagged a finger in front of us. "I fully intend to see that you're both severely reprimanded for this disgraceful conduct."

Sheila squeezed my hand. I knew by her gesture that we shared the same thoughts about this incident. Our head-nurse was stretching the whole thing out of proportion.

Yes, we put restraints on Mr. Bagsley, "Sheila said curtly. "We did it because he continuously climbed out of his bed, and we'd found him several times on the floor. This disturbed the other patients who shared his room and they had not been able to get any sleep with all the ruckus he had made.

"That's right, " I said, looking straight at Mrs. Brent.

Once we had resorted to this measure, "I added, " all of them slept peacefully including him. Sheila and I went in every two hours to reposition Mr. Bagsley. We untied him provided good skin care to avoid any breakdown before replacing the straps."

The disgusted look on Mrs. Brent's face told me that it did not matter what either of us said about giving Mr.Bagsley good nursing care. The oversight of not undoing the restraints before we had left the ward was going to get us both into a heap of trouble.

"I've already made out my report, " Mrs. Brent said. "This will be sent to the Director of Nursing and you will be notified when she will see you both." She waved a couple of sheets of paper in the air.

She glared at us. "I do not expect to come in tomorrow and find anymore problems as this. Do you both understand?"

"Yes, Mrs. Brent, " we both muttered.

"Well, " she said, as she marched away from the desk. " I hope you do for everyone's sake."

That night we still had to restrain this patient, but we made absolutely certain that before morning he was free. There was no other way the nursing staff on that unit could manage him.

We both got a reprimand from the Director of Nursing but she wasn't as upset about our actions as had been Mrs. Brent. The Director was more concerned with the fact that this man could have seriously injured himself had he fallen out of bed too many times. This had been part of our reasoning. We in no way had, at any time, meant him any harm.

Wanting to Look Nice

Mrs. White had been a resident of the chronic care facility for several years. She was not able to do anything for herself. She could talk, and sometimes she would do this incessantly.

The first time I met her, she told me she only liked being called by her married name. I too preferred that form of address especially by people who did not know me well or by someone much younger than me.

Mrs. White was quite happy to be lifted out of bed by the special lift. She sat in her chair most of the day except when we needed to return her to bed. She was a most pleasant person.

Mrs. White did not get very many visitors, but even this had no affect on her cheery nature, as she enjoyed talking with anyone who stopped by her chair. Mrs. White had several daughters but only one lived in the city.

This elderly lady enjoyed going down to the Sunday service held in the auditorium. She would always remind whoever was her caregiver that day that she needed to be ready in plenty of time for that outing.

The way our assignments worked was we had the same patients for a month so there would be some consistency of care. This also enabled the patient time to get to know us better.

I had noticed that Mrs. White had very few clothes. The ones that she had were all old and worn. She had said many times, "that she really wished her family would buy her some new ones."

The first weekend I was assigned to Mrs. White I went through her closet looking for something nice for her to wear to the service. It was going to be a special occasion and she wanted to look her best.

There wasn't anything suitable. I even went down to the hospital laundry thinking that I might find something there for her. We had quite a pile of clothes that families had left after their relatives had passed on. But there was nothing in her size. Now what?

"Were you able to find me something, " Mrs. White asked. Her oval lined face looked sad.

"No I'm really sorry, but there was nothing in your size." I patted her hand.

Here, though, let me take another look in your cupboard. There might something that we can fix."

Again I moved her dresses along the track and scanned each one. "Damn! Damn! Damn!" I mumbled under my breath. There wasn't anything even half-decent amongst them.

Just then, I spotted a box away up on the top shelf. I didn't know why I had missed it earlier. Standing on tiptoes I reached up and brought it down and out of the cupboard.

"What have you got there?" Mrs. White asked, as I placed the box on her bed.

"I don't know, "I said, "but let's take a look see, shall we."

I undid the string that held the lid shut. My patient anxiously was watching my every move.

"Wow!" my loud exclamation startled Mrs. White. She let out a small gasp. Inside the box was a brand new outfit in a gorgeous shade of blue.

Mrs. White's, brown eyes opened wide with astonishment. "Oh! My, "she murmured, "whose is that?"

"As far as I know, it must be yours. It was in your cupboard and look here, it's your size." I moved the tag so she could see it.

"It's so lovely, "she cooed." Her gnarled fingers gently touched the material.

"Well there's one thing for sure," I said, "you'll be the best-dressed lady in the building on Sunday. I'll just hang it up until then so these few creases will fall out."

Mrs. White released the dress and I placed it on a hanger in her closet. She looked as happy about the find as I felt inside because now at last she had something nice to wear.

Working in a chronic care facility requires a special type of nursing. It is more challenging in some ways because one becomes more attached to the patients. There is not the constant turnover of patients that one has in an acute care setting. The extra challenge always for me was not to let their problems and frustrations become mine.

I was not good at avoiding some involvement in how they were feeling. However, had I been different I would not have got to share their experiences as fully as I did.

Sunday morning ablutions for Mrs. White were a time of absolute excitement. She was barely able to control herself as I brought out the blue dress from her closet.

"Oh! It's so lovely. I haven't had anything that was as pretty as that. Do you think it's pretty Nurse?"

Yes, Mrs. White, " I smiled, "I do, and you will look stunning in it." I had already partially dressed her. All that remained was to get her into the dress. With her cooperation I slid it carefully over her head and worked it down her torso.

"Oh! It is so nice; it feels so soft. Do you think it is made of silk?

"I don't know. Anyway the color looks lovely on you and it fits you beautifully."

I smiled at the happy look on her face. " I'll just go and get the Hoyer lift, a special device we used to transfer immobile patients. I will get another nurse to help me.

Walking out into the hallway, I met Nancy, a nurse's aide, and she agreed to assist me.

"Oh my, " Nancy moved toward Mrs. White's bed. "Don't you look smart today."

"Where did you find this outfit?" Nancy quizzed me.

"It was in her cupboard in a box stuck away at the back on the top shelf." I replied, " anyway don't you think she looks sharp in it?"

"I certainly do." Nancy said smiling. "Now, Mrs. White, lets get this behind you without getting your new outfit creased." Getting my patient up in her chair was easy with the lift and my peers help.

"Now," I said to Mrs. White, "let's do your hair and maybe we can find a little rouge as well for your cheeks."

I took her brush from the dresser drawer and started to tidy her unruly grey mop. She had natural curls and they were in disarray from her lying in bed.

"My goodness Mrs. White don't you look grand today." The head nurse said. I had moved my patient out into the foyer ready to go down to the auditorium. She came over and looked closely at the blue dress.

"Who's been buying you such a nice outfit?"

"I don't know, " said Mrs. White, " but it is lovely isn't it?"

The other staff members and some of Mrs. Whites friends all agreed that she did indeed look delightful. The big smile and the happy expression on my patient's face were most rewarding. My warm feeling was to be short-lived. Mrs. White's daughter had decided that she was going to visit her mother on this special Sunday. For me it became a day that I'll never forget.

The church service was over and Mrs. White was sitting in her room having a little afternoon refreshment. She had already filled me in on all that had taken placed downstairs. Her happiness was intense. Her face glowed.

Then her daughter marched into the room.

For a brief moment, she glanced at her mother. There was no greeting, no hello.

"Where? Who?" She screamed. "What the hell are you doing in that dress?"

Instantly Mrs. White's composure changed and she looked at me with tears beginning to trickle down her face.

"Excuse me, " I confronted my patients angry daughter, "what do you think your doing coming in here and upsetting your mother like that? You have no right to speak to her in that way." Now my tone matched hers.

"We'll see who has the right here, " she yelled, as she flounced out of the room.

"Oh my goodness what have I done to upset her so?" The tears now turned into a flood and Mrs. White began to sob.

"You've done absolutely nothing wrong." I said, placing my arm around her shoulder.

"It's obvious there's some sort of a dispute with your daughter but I have no idea what it is. Anyway, lets not worry about it. It's going to be alright." I held her close as she gradually quieted down.

"You're sure? " she looked anxiously at me.

"I'm sure, " I told her as I started to dry her tears with a face cloth.

Mrs. White's daughter strode back into the room. On seeing her my patient cringed and tried to avoid looking at her.

"You," she grabbed my arm, "are to go to the Nursing Supervisor's office immediately. That's at once, do you hear."

"I'm not deaf. Yes I heard you." I moved her hand away.

"You can just leave that for me to do." She snatched the cloth from my hand and started to rub it briskly over her mother's face.

"Please don't leave me Nurse, I've got nothing to say to my daughter, " The elderly woman said, her voice trembling.

"Well I've got some things to say to you Mother. And your nurse is going to find out that she's made a big mistake crossing with me."

"Mrs. White," I said smiling to try to reassure her. "I promise I won't be long. It'll be fine."

Unfortunately, not everything was fine as I found out when I entered the supervisor's office.

"Mrs. Stirling, " she said sternly, "I've had Mrs. Whites daughter in here to see me. It seems you've done something that has really upset her. " Her tone told me clearly she wasn't pleased by all of this.

"I don't understand what it is that I've done, " I replied.

"Did you or did you not take a box out of her mother's cupboard that held a brand new outfit?"

I nodded, "Yes, yes I did."

"And did you put this dress on Mrs. White and is she in fact still wearing it?"

"Yes, but what on earth is wrong with that?" I retorted.

"I don't know if you are aware of it but this lady has nothing decent to wear. Her clothes are an utter disgrace." I glanced at my supervisor's face.

"All Mrs. White wanted was something nice to put on to go to church. When I discovered that box with that lovely dress in it why wouldn't I have put it on her?"

"Because, Mrs. Stirling," she sat unsmiling, "that dress is the one she is to wear when she is laid out."

I could not believe what I was hearing.

"Let me see if I have got this right?" I said with disbelief. "Mrs. White has a brand new outfit which is only to be worn once she is dead, and while she's living it doesn't matter what she looks like?"

"Mrs. Stirling, " the voice seemed softer, "maybe in England your customs are a little different from ours. But yes that outfit that you've put on your patient today is her funeral clothes."

"Miss Knight," I said aghast. " you're right I've never ever heard such an awful thing. It looks as if I have a lot to learn about your customs. Yet, I cannot believe this is a normal behavior. At least I really hope it isn't."

"Well, " Miss Knight said," when you undress Mrs. White later you will put that dress back in the box and that will be the end of it." Her displeasure about this affair was evident by the grim look on her face.

I was angry. Angry that any daughter could be so callous to buy her mother a new outfit for her funeral but without giving her anything decent to wear while she was alive.

"I cannot believe you agree with this, " I looked straight into my supervisor's eyes.

"It's not always what I believe or want but what the resident's family wants and demands we do, " she said.

For once I was at a loss what to say to the woman who sat opposite me. All I was certain about was that dress was going to be worn by that elderly lady more often than her daughter had ever intended it to be. Even now when I recall that incident it leaves me wondering about some people's priorities.

Returning to Mrs. White's room, I found her alone.

"Has your daughter gone Mrs. White?"

"Yes, " she said. "I hope you didn't get into any trouble."

"Not a bit, " I said, " as I told you everything is just fine. Now about this dress we'll keep it for your Sunday best, if that's okay with you?"

The round, kindly face smiled, as she nodded her approval. That's exactly what we did with it.

Strangely enough nothing, more was ever said to me about this incident. I like to think that maybe the supervisor had informed the daughter that her mother's clothes were in need of some attention. All I remember is that outfit gave a little old lady a great deal of enjoyment while she was living, and that was all that mattered to me.

Poetic Justice does Happen

"My name, " the short, stout man muttered, "is Mr. Grilali, and you can get my wife checked in right away. He pushed a slim, small figure up to the desk. "I do not have a lot of time to waste; I'm a very busy man"

There were several of us working in, and around the nurse's station, and we all watched this man's conduct with astonishment. I felt sorry for his wife, because he did not seem to care how she felt.

I looked straight at him and said. "If you just go down the north hall, " I pointed to the hallway, I will be right in to see you." I looked right at Mrs. Grilali, but she made no indication that she had heard me or understood.

"Just don't be long in coming, because the sooner you get my wife fixed up the better it'll be for me. Mr. Grilali, turned and hurriedly propelled his wife towards her room.

"Wow!" I said aloud. "I wonder what his problem is?"

Several of my peers chuckled, and nodded their heads in agreement.

"Finally, " Mr. Grilali muttered crossly, when I appeared. "You certainly took your time coming."

Choosing to ignore him, I turned and spoke to his wife. "I need to ask you a few questions, if that's alright with you?"

"She isn't capable of answering anything, " he said scowling at me. "I'll tell you all you need to know."

"Mr. Grilali, " I said looking him straight in the eye. "Just who is the patient?"

"There's no need to speak to me like that." He glared angrily. You know quite well it's my wife who is coming in here. She has some sort of women's problem and that's why we haven't been able to produce any children."

"Then I'd appreciate it if you would keep quiet while your wife and I get her history done."

"You western women have no respect for your men, and it shows in the way you treat them. Just do what you have to do, but I'm not leaving the room." He moved over to a chair and sat down.

Mrs. Grilali was sitting on the edge of the bed, with her head down and her hands tightly clasped in her lap.

I touched her gently on the shoulder. "I see your first name is Rosa, do you mind if I call you that?'

She looked up nodded and smiled.

I smiled. "I see that you're in for some tests. The doctor will explain these in detail to you when he comes in to see you, once I'm through with my paperwork."

"Now look here,you. " Mr. Grilali barked. "I want to see the doctor when he comes in to see my wife. "I want to know exactly what he is going to do so I can get the son I want."

"That shouldn't be a problem." I said.

" He took a deep breath, " even if it is, that is the way, I am going to have it."

Even with many noisy interruptions from her husband, I finally got Rosa's paper work completed.

"I'll leave you now." I said to her. The doctor should soon be in to see you."

Mr. Grilali came and stood right in front of me. He sneered. "You'd better tell him to hurry up. I do not enjoy waiting for anyone."

Biting back an urge to make a snide remark, I moved around him and quickly left the room.

The young intern was waiting to see my history before going down to see this couple. As he took them from me I felt I had to warn him. "You had better watch out for this lady's husband he's awfully demanding."

"Thanks nurse, " he said. "I'll be on my guard."

When the young doctor returned to the desk, I was busy charting. I noticed that his usual pleasant face now wore a scowl.

146

He gave me a quick glance as he sat down across from me. "Well, you were right that man is certainly something else. When I suggested to him that the fertility problem might be his, and related to his sperm count, he went up one side of me and came down the other."

I smiled. "Oh! Yes I can well imagine how he'd respond to such an idea. His masculinity being challenged would not sit well with him at all."

The young boyish face grinned. "Well even if he doesn't want to think about it that's a strong possibility. It could well be the answer why his wife hasn't conceived."

When I next went in to check on Mrs. Grilali, she was conversing with someone on the telephone. She motioned to me to wait until she was finished.

I looked with some astonishment at the change in her. Gone was the timid looking wife and in her place was this seemingly vivacious woman.

"It's alright nurse I'm just talking with my friend. She comes from the same part of Italy that I do. We've known each other a long time."

"That's okay." I said. "I only wanted to see how you were settling in, and if you needed anything."

"No thank-you nurse, I'm fine." She resumed her conversation with her caller.

Over the course of the following few days Rosa underwent several tests She took them all calmly and never complained once. Her husband on the other hand had fast become the most unwelcome sight on the ward. He constantly berated everyone. He did not think the hospital was doing enough to help his wife.

What I remember more vividly was the day when all the reports were in on this case. The same young intern who had admitted Mrs. Grilali was in the nurse's station going through all the test results.

Suddenly, he let out a loud laugh. "I knew it. I knew it."

There were several of us close by, and we all looked in his direction. Again, he laughed aloud.

"What is it?" I asked.

"There's absolutely nothing wrong with Mrs. Grilali. She is capable of conceiving at any time, so it is her husband."

I raised my eyebrows as I peered at him. "Well, there's one thing for sure, I don't envy the job of the person who has to tell him this."

"Em...Yes, I know what you mean. He frowned. "I guess that will be my chore. But you know, in a way I'm going to enjoy it. This man has done nothing but run down everyone and everything about this hospital. His ego could stand a bit of deflating."

"Yes, I do agree with you." I said. "As long as he doesn't end up taking it out on his wife. Somehow, I just can't see him accepting your news well."

I could not have been more right about Mr. Grilali not taking it well. When he was given the results of his wife's tests he promptly marched down to the desk.

"I demand to see the person in charge of this hospital." He stormed. I have some serious complaints I want them to hear."

The head nurse, Miss Wells, who had felt the lash of this man's tongue on several occasions, looked up from where she sat. "What is it you want Mr.Grilali? Perhaps I can help you?"

"These test results are not right. My wife cannot bear children because she has a problem with her productive organs. That's why I brought her here to have them fixed."

"I see." Miss Wells muttered. "And, what do you want the Chief Executive Officer of this hospital to do?" She was now standing facing this man.

"I'd like them to be all done over again." He yelled.

"I'm sorry that you're not pleased with the reports of your wife's tests." She said. "But to do them all over again is out of the question."

Angrily Mr. Grilali turned away from the desk, and stomped back down the hall.

There were several of us who could not help smiling at this turn of events. Even though in a way I felt sorry for him, I also

148

thought that it was irony the way it had turned out. I just hoped that Rosa wouldn't suffer because of it.

Mr. Grilali had his wife immediately discharged once he knew that nothing else would be done, so I was not able to assess his manner towards her. Recalling this incident again has prompted me to wonder how, and if, they ever resolved his fertility problem, and if she bore him a son.

The Call of the Night

To have a restful sleep is the goal of most of us. To be able to do this as a patient in a hospital isn't always an option.

Mr. Cooper was a large, obese man who had come in to hospital to see why he was having a disturbance in his breathing pattern. As I hadn't been on night duty while he'd been a patient before I had no inkling of his other major problem.

He was an affable man and had undergone the numerous tests well. He told me, " I've got to find out why this is happening because both my wife and I are beginning to get worried."

"I can understand that Mr. Cooper, "I said. " When anyone's breathing stops their brain cells get most upset." I smiled. "It's not a highly recommended practice."

He laughed aloud. "I like that. I can just see all those little cells frantically running around wondering why their air supply has suddenly been shut off."

I laughed with him. "That's quite an amusing picture you've got their, Mr. Cooper, " I said. "You've got a great sense of humor."

He grinned. "Well I try. At my age there's not a lot I can do except keep myself cheerful."

He winked cheekily. "Mind you I can still think about other things I used to be able to do even if I can't actually do any of them now."

"Okay," I said. "We seem to be drifting off the topic here. Why do you think you're having this problem with your breathing?"

"You know it's really an odd thing," he said. "During the day it doesn't seem to bother me as much as it does through the night. Now I wonder, nurse why that is?"

150

I was soon to find out.

The other nurse on duty and I had just gotten everyone on the ward settled down for the night. We were seated at the desk checking some of the patient's charts when we heard this dreadful noise.

I looked up and glanced over at her. She raised her eyebrows at me and shook her head.

"What in blazes is that all about?" I said to her.

It was as though the same question had come to many of the other patients on the ward. The call buttons started to light up in large numbers. When we asked what was needed all we were told was, "Do something about that awful noise."

I shrugged my shoulders. "Guess we'd better go and find the person who's responsible for waking everyone else up."

"You go," she told me. "Just follow the sounds."

As I made my way down the hall several irate faces appeared at the doors of their rooms."

"What is all that racket?" one patient said.

"Sounds like a bull in heat, " were another man's comments.

"Well I don't care what or who it is. Just go and shut him up, " I was ordered.

As I had half way suspected, Mr. Cooper was the person creating the furor on the ward. I found this gentleman lying on his back and snoring so loudly, I was astonished that he had not woken himself up.

I gently shook him to try to waken him. He was completely oblivious of the noise he was making. I smiled to myself as I tried to rouse him. I thought, how difficult it must be for Mr. Cooper's wife trying to get any rest.

"What? What? What is it?" He drowsily asked.

I smiled. "You sir, are making enough noise with your snoring that you've got everyone else on the ward in a fit."

"Who me?" Mr. Cooper said with disbelief.

I nodded, "Yes, you sir"

"No, no it can't be. Must be someone else." He shook his head, "I know I snore a little bit but it's not what I would call any great noise."

It took a bit of tactful persuasion to convince this pleasant elderly man that his snoring was indeed a real dilemma. It was decided to keep the door of his room closed at night. He was assured that the nursing staff would be checking on him frequently and if he needed anything he just had to use his call-bell.

Mr. Cooper's snoring was at the root of his breathing problem. He underwent minor surgery to correct this and it improved things for him and his wife.

I have never, however, after or since ever heard anyone who could come close to making the noise that this man made when he was asleep. It was truly unique.

The Truth couldn't be Told

I stood transfixed by the sight before my eyes. I could hardly believe the extent of what I was looking at.

"How does it look nurse?" my elderly patient asked anxiously.

The teacher had removed the initial dressing. It was my task with her supervision to clean and redress this wound. I could see just by glancing at it this was going to be a mammoth task. My initial reaction was that I was not capable enough to do it, but neither my teacher nor my patient shared my feelings. Both of them waited patiently for me to begin.

Mrs. Victor was a petite, elderly woman. My first meeting with her had been on her entry to the surgical unit.

"I don't think I have anything to worry about, " she'd told me. "I'm sure that my GP is being overly cautious sending me here."

She had been having some serious vaginal bleeding. The Pap smear that she had finally allowed her doctor to perform had shown she had Cancer. All of this was clearly written up in the reports we had received.

I was curious why she had not ever had a Pap smear before this first one. "Was there some reason why you had never had this done before?" I asked.

I remember she gave me the sweetest smile and said. " Why yes dear. It's not something that nice ladies allow their doctors to do to them."

"Excuse me, " I said. "You think that it is not right to protect yourself. It only takes a few minutes in a doctor's office."

"Now, nurse I didn't say that, " she smiled again. "What I said was that it is not something that a single lady as I am, would agree to. It's just not proper."

Because of her misguided attitude, this woman now faced major surgery. Yet she still seemed to think that what she had believed was correct.

I wondered how many women of Mrs. Victor's age thought the same way. I was dismayed to learn later, from some research figures, that the number of women who thought like her in the 1970's was high.

This patient had to undergo numerous examinations by many doctors and specialists. I thought it was ironic that this lady had refused to have Pap smears because she felt it wasn't right, and now she had all these people daily checking these very same personal areas she'd aimed to keep private. I was sure that it must have been difficult for her.

Mrs. Victor seemed to cope better than I expected with this situation. She never protested and when she was asked, "How are you doing?" she'd always smile and say, "Just fine. Thank-you very much for asking."

The surgical team had decided on a procedure that would remove all the cancerous cells at once. The doctors appeared confident that Mrs. Victor would be fine afterwards. She should be well enough to return home.

As she was my patient, I had the task of prepping her for this surgery. I tried to complete this task as discreetly as possible.

She astonished me by saying, "It's all right nurse. Just do what you have to do. I know now that I've been a foolish woman. I should have let my doctor give me those Pap tests as he had so often suggested."

Mrs. Victor sighed deeply. "If I'd only known then what I know now."

This was one of those times when nothing I might have said would help. I kept quiet, and I carried on with what I was doing.

The next day I saw her off to the operating room. I wished her the best of luck and that everything would go well. She squeezed my hand and drowsily said, "Thank-you nurse. I'll be just fine."

The following day she was again my patient. Now here I was in her room to perform a dressing change. My stomach was in a knot as I tried not to let this dear lady see that I found her wound mind-boggling. I'd never seen anything like it ever before and I really didn't know where to begin.

By using the strict aseptic measures, I had been taught I prepared myself to carry out this procedure. I was extremely grateful that I had a mask on because it helped to hide some of my face from Mrs. Victor's view. I didn't want her to see how I felt nor frighten her in any way.

"How does it look nurse?" she asked me again.

I looked into my supervisor's eyes and non-verbally asked her by raising my eyebrows, what reply should I give this lady.

My teacher shook her head. I knew that we could not tell Mrs. Victor the truth but she needed to be told something.

Taking a deep breath I swallowed hard and said. "It's early yet. The wound is still fresh from the operation so the healing process hasn't really started."

Mrs. Victor smiled at us. "I could have saved myself all of this misery you know, if I had heeded my family doctors suggestions. I'm glad it's now all over."

This elderly lady lived only a few days after that. Before then, she spoke to me several times of her regret that she had not listened to her physician. However, she blamed no one but herself for what she had had to suffer.

Given Another Chance

"I don't think I'm ever going to get better, " Pat said. Her hazel eyes peered apprehensive at me. In her late twenties she was back on the respiratory ward because of her ongoing problem with chronic obstructive lung disease.

"Now the Doctors are telling me I might be a good candidate for a lung transplant." She shook her head. "I don't know about something as that; we're talking major, major surgery."

"Yes, " I said, "you're right, that is a serious procedure but what's the alternative?"

Pats round plump face shone with perspiration. She fiddled with the nasal prongs that gave her the additional oxygen she had to have on all the time.

"My nose feels sore, " she said. "Would you look at it."

Pat started to hyperventilate while I looked at the tubing.

"Just try and slow your breathing down Pat, " I coaxed her. "I'll have this fixed for you in just a few minutes."

After I had replaced the prongs back in her nostrils, she sighed and lay back in bed. "What alternative do I have? I know I can't go on much longer like this, I'm getting so tired."

Sitting on the edge of her bed, I asked. "What else did the team tell you about having a transplant?"

"They told me that I would have to have both of my lungs replaced. Then I'd be on a special medication for the rest of my life. This would be to make sure that my body didn't reject the new organs."

"You've been taking medication for most of your life anyway," I said, "so that shouldn't be too difficult."

She smiled wearily. "Yes that's true, but it's the thought of being out for all those hours. That's what's frightening."

156

I gently placed my hand over hers. "Have to tell you, you're looking at a nurse who is a complete coward when it comes to anything like that. In fact I've got a enormous streak of yellow running all the way down my back"

Pat laughed. "Oh! I don't think so. How could you be a nurse if you were that scared?"

"Quite easily, " I smiled. "I can help anyone who's going for any form of treatment. Just as long as it's not me that's having it done"

She laughed. "I get your point. Yes, I guess that I could do that as well." She frowned, "But I still don't know if I can face going through a transplant."

"Look, " I said. "I have other patients to see, so I have to leave. You lie here and give it some more thought, and I'll be back later to see what you think."

Checking that she had everything she needed I headed back down to the desk. I didn't envy Pat. The decision she was being asked to make was one I knew I wouldn't want to have to face. I knew, however, that she had to get treatment soon for her health condition.

Pat had a male friend and I knew their relationship was serious. She had told me that ideally she would love to get married, but having a debilitating disease had prevented that. I hoped she might think about this when trying to figure out what to do.

After talking it over with her friend and family, Pat made up her mind to go with the doctor's plan. Once the special team was informed, the preparation procedure swung into action. There was a lot of work to be done getting Pat ready and she took most of it well.

To get an exact match for her she had to be picked many times for blood work, which did get to her after awhile. I remember her saying, " I feel a bit like a pin cushion that's run out of space."

Her close friend Terry came in often to give her moral support, which was a great help. As soon as the team had all the data they needed Pat was sent home to wait for a donor.

Transplant patients have many times said, "the waiting is much worse than going through the actual surgery. Never knowing if there will be a matching donor found is highly stressful."

Pat was lucky. Her match was found within a few weeks. She was re-admitted to our floor for the surgery.

All the staff who knew Pat over her many admissions was as pent up as she was. The tension and emotional high in and around her room was at a fever pitch.

This feeling increased even more when we learned that the surgeons had determined that they would not only give Pat two new lungs but another heart as well. This would be the first time that this procedure had ever been performed at this hospital. It was an exciting time to be working on that ward.

Pat took this added news well. "All I want is an opportunity to live as normal a life as I'm able, " she said. "I know this will give me a good chance to do that."

Before she went down to the operating room, many of the floor staff wished her well. "We'll all be waiting for you to come back to us, " we told her.

"Pat, see you don't drag out your stay in the coronary care unit, " I said teasingly. "We expect to see you up and about as never before." I looked at Terry's concerned face now almost touching Pats. "Isn't that right?" I asked him.

He looked up and smiled at the group of concerned staff members clustered around Pat's stretcher. "Yes that's the whole purpose of this. So she will be able to chase me instead of me running all the time after her."

After a final emotional goodbye, she was transported down to the OR. Pat did not immediately return to our ward but when she did the change in her health status was astonishing. She was able to function with only a little additional oxygen therapy; eventually this was discontinued altogether.

Her activity level had doubled and it was not long before she and Terry started to plan their wedding. Some of the younger staff members were able to attend this happy event.

We all got to see the photographs and from the glowing look on both the bride and grooms faces it was evident that the decision to have the transplant had been the right one. An unknown family's selfless generosity had given Pat the second chance that she had so desperately needed. I was fortunate to share part of this major event in her life.

When does Caring Cease?

"You definitely have an over powering maternal instinct." Dr. Blake said sarcastically.

I looked with amazement at him. "I've never been accused of that before, " I said.

"Well," he said firmly, " believe me you do have that problem. I personally think it could be a real hindrance to you as a nurse."

Being a mature student in the Registered Nurse's program this doctor's attack on my method of caring for my patient hurt. I'd always thought part of a nurse's role was to see that a patient had proper follow up when being discharged. I didn't think we were supposed to just put them out on the street.

This conversation was taking place because I had wanted to help one my male patient find a place that would take him in. It was obvious from the doctor's remarks that he and I did not share the same opinion of what we should do.

"So, tell me what do you think we should do with Mr. Brent?" Doctor Blake's full face closely scrutinized mine.

I gulped nervously and took a deep breath, "I think we should make sure he has a place to go to before we discharge him. That would be the right thing to do."

Dr. Blake let out a loud laugh. "Oh! You do, do you? And just where do you think we are going to get a place that will take him?"

Now, thoroughly irate, but knowing I daren't let this doctor see that, I gritted my teeth. " I know that there are several very good halfway houses in the city, I'm sure that anyone of them would be only too pleased to take Mr. Brent."

Doctor Blake grinned. "I must say, you seem to have got this all figured out. Maybe you should check with the patient first and see what he wants to do."

As he moved, away from the nurse's station he muttered, " If the patient is agreeable you can do what ever you want. All I know is one way or another Mr. Brent is being discharged out of here today."

Mr. Brent was a middle-aged man who had come to the hospital suffering from the effects of years of alcoholic abuse. He had no relatives, no friends, and no permanent address. While I had been providing him with his care I'd found him to be a fairly pleasant man who was finally able to admit that he was an alcoholic.

"I do not blame anyone else for my poor health, " he told me. "It's all my own fault."

"Being able to recognize that is the first step in dealing with it, "I said.

"Yes, I guess you're right, but it doesn't do me much good now does it?" He shrugged his shoulders.

"The docs have told me my liver is shot so that's a bummer."

"Yes, Mr. Brent you're right that's not something one wants to hear." I said, but on another subject, how do you feel about being discharged out of here today?"

His gaunt, pinched face looked anxious, " I've got no place to go. Are they going to just put me out on the street?"

"That's what I needed to ask you about. Where, would you go?"

I inclined my head. "You've told me that you don't have anywhere to live. I thought I would see if one of the halfway houses in this city would take you in. That's if you think it's alright."

"That would be great nurse, " he smiled, " I wouldn't be any trouble. You can assure them of that."

"I'm sure you won't be any bother." I said, " Anyway, the people who run these establishments are professionals. They would know how to help you even if something did happen."

I checked with my instructor first before making the call. She agreed that it would be inhumane to release Mr. Brent without first finding him a place to stay.

The second halfway house that I called was willing to take Mr. Brent. They told me that a social worker would come to the hospital and pick him up.

Just before he left the ward Mr. Brent came to the desk and asked to see me.

Smiling broadly he said, " Thanks for all your kindness. You are going to make a very good nurse. You really do care about people."

He had no idea how much I needed to hear that. So before waving him goodbye I gave him a big hug, which he immediately returned. I knew that I had done the right thing in helping this man. What Dr. Blake thought no longer concerned me.

Nothing but Flowers

"He never, ever, comes to see me." Mrs. Glover's voice trembled.

"He was so caring when he was younger." The tears flowed and she sobbed.

Placing my arm around her shoulders, I stood quietly by her side.

A nurse is called to act in a wide and varied number of situations for his/her patients. They are trained to administer analgesics; to ease physical pain, but sometimes trying to lessen a person's mental anguish can be much more difficult.

Mrs. Glover had come to the medical floor for an assessment of an internal problem. She had undergone several tests, but had no definite diagnosis. On top of everything else, this was causing her some concerns.

On her admission to the floor, she had told me that her son Lawrence was her only living relative. She said that over the last six years she had only spoken to him on the telephone. She thought that this was partly due to his being such a busy person.

"But, you know he's always sending me gorgeous flowers." She said.

Mrs. Glover enjoyed telling me about Lawrence's accomplishments. "He worked hard and put himself through University, " she said. "And now he's a successful businessman with his own company."

It was obvious she was proud of him. Still, I couldn't help wondering why he never visited her.

"What does your son say when you ask him to come and see you?" I asked.

"Oh, I'd never ask him to do that. He'd be very annoyed with me if I did."

"Why would he be annoyed with you? Maybe, he thinks you don't want to see him. That is possible you know."

"Oh, that's not true. More than anything else I want him to visit me. I really miss him." Mrs. Glover's face turned pale.

I touched her hand, and looked closely into her blue eyes. "Well, perhaps what you need to do is tell him how much he means to you. What about telling him that what you would like more than anything else is to see him."

"But.....But...we have never." She shook her head. "Nurse, I just don't know if I could say that. I'm afraid it might make things worse." Tears again welled and spilled.

"I can't see how it would make your relationship worse." I said, offering her a Kleenex. "Sometimes we have to be a little more honest about how we feel, with those we love. We mother's often assume that our children know how we feel."

"Yes, I know what you say is right but it's not always easy to do." She rubbed the tissue briskly across her face.

A volunteer suddenly appeared carrying a beautiful bouquet of flowers.

"Mrs. Glover, " she said, " these are for you." She placed the lovely arrangement in my patient's arms.

"You see nurse." Mrs. Glover let out another loud sob. "You see, once again he has only sent me flowers. I really don't want them, I'd much rather he had come."

"I think, after what you've told me, that the only way that is going to happen is for you ask him to come. If that's something you cannot do yourself, I could get someone from the social services department to do it for you."

"No! No! I'll do it, I'll do it. "Mrs. Glover declared. "Anyway, I know Lawrence would get furious if I had someone else telephoning him about this. I'm sure of that."

"You just let me know if you change your mind." I smiled. "The social workers that we have here are very adept at talking with family members."

She nodded and returned my smile. "You're most kind. And, why don't I give you these to put out at the nurses station, then more people will be able to see them." She deftly handed me the bouquet.

"Well if you're sure you don't want them?" I said.

"Look at all I've got now in my room. I don't need anymore." She pointed at the vases of flowers.

"Yes, you do have quite a display, don't you. Your son is very generous."

"I suppose you could say that." She softly mumbled.

"He probably didn't choose them." Mrs. Glover gave a deep sigh. "I don't know if he even ordered them."

"Lawrence has several secretaries, and one of them probably did it for him." There was a tremble again in her voice.

Attempting to change her downcast mood, I smiled.

"Are you certain you want us to have these? They really are beautiful, and they smell wonderful.

"Yes, I'm quite sure." She brushed them away with her hands as I picked the bouquet up.

"Thanks a lot!" I said. "I'll put them up on the top of the desk so everyone can enjoy them. I am sure that they will cheer many people. Thank-you again Mrs. Glover."

"No thank-you nurse." She said. "You've given me a lot to think about regarding my relationship with my son, and you've taken the time to listen to a foolish old lady's ranting."

I shook my head and smiled. "No problem. It is all part of our job description, to listen to our patients. And, I don't see you at all as being a foolish old lady."

Her brown eyes twinkled. "That's kind of you to say that. Now, if you don't mind I think I'll take a little rest."

I helped Mrs. Glover get her settled in bed, and left her lying listening to a tape of her favorite music. She seemed to be a lot more relaxed.

Everyone on the ward who saw the flower arrangement commented on them. I wondered how much they had cost my patient's son, because they were beautiful

I would like to be able to say that Lawrence came in to see his mother while she was on our ward, but he didn't. She told me later that she had called him. Moreover, as I had suggested, she had told him how much she longed to see him, and what a visit from him meant to her. After we had had this conversation, she only spent a few more days in hospital.

Before leaving Mrs. Glover said, "She was confident that Lawrence would eventually come and see her. He was a good son."

I have always hoped that they did finally get together. The steady stream of flowers, and the telephone calls, was no substitute for that personal contact that she wanted to have with him. I related to this incident not just as a nurse but also as a mother.

The Secret to Life

"Yes, I believe I understand now." Paul's, young face looked tired. His soft, blue eyes were sunken and rimmed with dark circles. In spite of that, I was pleased to see that the angry glare they had had earlier was missing.

Paul had arrived on the ward full of energy and excited about being newly engaged. "This is my very own special girl, nurse, " he had said as he introduced Susan to me. The fact he was being hospitalized for an investigation of a questionable mole on his back hadn't dampened his happy demeanor.

He knew that he was going to have to face a barrage of tests but as he said, " They shouldn't be too bad. I'm sure that this little lump isn't anything to worry about."

While I was completing his admission Susan was sitting beside him. They held hands. Paul leant over frequently and gently kissed his fiancée. It did make getting his documentation awkward, but I didn't mind. I had a feeling that he needed to have her as support.

Before Susan left, they were seen later embracing by the elevator. As he came back past the desk, this friendly young man gave me a saucy wink and said, "What do you think of my girl, nurse? She is going to make a super wife. Do you agree?" He beamed. "I'm a real lucky fellow."

I nodded my head and smiled while Paul jauntily walked back to his room. I hoped that the lump he had would prove to be nothing for both of their sakes.

Paul under went several days of tests as well as a biopsy. He had to wait for all the results but his attitude was still cheerful. Susan came in every day to see him. We tried to ensure that they had plenty of time to be alone.

When all the findings had been compiled, they were placed in Paul's chart. As I read them, I felt a terrible sorrow. Nurses often ask, " why do such things have to happen?" Although we know that there is no concrete answer. I silently asked that question now as I read this young man's diagnosis.

The next day the specialist went in to see this man. When he came back out of the room he asked." Who has Paul Jacobs as their patient?"

I owned up that I was his nurse. "I think you should go in and see him." He said.

"You need to reassure that young man that we are going to do everything we can for him." He shrugged his shoulders. "At the moment he doesn't want to believe anything I've told him."

I knew somehow that this was not going to be easy. I nodded. "I'll go in and talk with him." I said.

Before entering Paul's room, I took a deep breath. I hoped that I would be able to face him in a professional manner.

Susan was sitting up close to Paul. They were locked in an embrace. Her oval, fair face was strained looking.

Going up to them, I placed my hand on Paul's arm. "I'm really very sorry to learn about your diagnosis."

Susan began to sob." It is just so unfair. What has Paul done to deserve this horrible thing?"

"I don't believe it works that way Susan," I softly said. Her blonde head turned and she glared at me. "Well just how does it work nurse?" she shouted." You must see a lot of people who come into the hospital with all kinds of problems. So you must know."

Paul tried to quiet his fiancée's ranting. "It's okay my love," he whispered." I know exactly what the problem is; they've got my biopsy results mixed up with someone else's."

Susan vigorously nodded her head. "That's got to be it, " she said excitedly." These things do happen don't they?" She stared at me, wanting me to confirm what he had said.

I looked into Paul's wan face, hoping to see a clue as to whether or not he really thought this was the truth. He quickly averted his eyes from my gaze and nuzzled Susan's neck.

"Look love you go and get some lunch." he kissed her. " I need to get something sorted out with my nurse."

"But I ...." Susan began to protest.

"Never mind the buts." he smiled. "You've not eaten anything today and I don't want you getting sick on me."

With reluctance, Susan did as he had ordered. "I won't be long, " she waved, as she headed out the door.

When we were alone Paul picked up the telephone. "I'd like you to phone the lab for me, " he said, " and ask them for my real biopsy results."

"What do you think they are going to say to that request?" I asked.

"How the hell would I know that," Paul growled. "All I do know is that this can't be happening to me." His eyes stared angrily as he strode up and down the room.

"Look, " I said, " if it's going to help you feel any better.............."

"Make me feel better, " he stormed." How can it do that?"

I shook my head. It was tragic to see this young man in so much distress. "I don't mind calling them for you, " I said.

"No! No! It's no good, " he said dejectedly. " I think I knew all the time, deep down, that this wasn't just a simple mole." "But dammit!, " he yelled. " Why did this have to happen now? My life is all coming together."

Paul sat down on the edge of his bed. For a few minutes he remained like that with his face covered by his hands.

"Look nurse," he stared into my face. "I'd appreciate it if you'd leave me alone for awhile. I really need to think this all out for myself."

I did as he wanted, but I could not help wondering just how he was going to come to terms with his diagnosis. Learning that one has malignant melanoma I knew from past experiences with patients does not come easy.

When later I went back into his room, the drapes were closed and he was lying on top of his bed. I was about to leave when he sat up and asked me to hear what he had decided.

"I've figured it all out, " he quietly told me, " it took me awhile but it is very simple really."

"What have you figured out Paul?" I searched his face for some sort of a clue.

His gaunt face briefly smiled. "The whole purpose to all of this, " he said. "I know what the secret is to life."

I watched him and waited expectantly to hear what he was going to say. It is something that I have never forgotten.

He gave a deep breath. "Well, it's like this nurse." He frowned. "It's all very simple. When we are born, we all are given the same amount of time. The thing is, some people never do anything so theirs just goes on and on until eventually they die. I've done so much in my few years that I've used up my quota." He tightened his lips together. "Which means, it's going to end long before I really want it to."

I was at a loss to know what to say. I thought what he had said was profound. I stood there not uttering anything.

He looked intently at me. "What do you think nurse? Am I right? Or am a away out in the left field?"

I shook my head. "I honestly don't know what to say, but if it eases the pain you're feeling then it's okay by me."

Paul left the hospital shortly after this for a brief while. He returned to us next as a married man. Sadly, soon after that, with his beloved Susan cradling him in her arms, he died.

Humor With a Twist

"That's not my baby, " the young, woman informed me, " it's hers." She pointed to one of the other new mums in the four-bed ward.

I freaked. My throat constricted and my stomach fluttered. What had I done? How could I have mixed the babies up? I had been so careful making sure that the right baby was deposited into the correct spot in the cart. Now all sorts of terrible thoughts raced through my mind as I moved across the room.

Working in the new baby nursery was one of my favorite areas. The babies were delightful.

It always amused me to see how the young fathers reacted when given the small bundle to carry for the first time. Most of them seemed to believe that their baby had to be treated like an eggshell. They held them as though they feared it might shatter into a million tiny pieces.

Every new baby was weighed, measured and bathed as soon as they came into the nursery. At the time of my nursing experience in this unit, we would place the babe's surname firmly on their back, using a piece of Elastoplast. This was done to make sure that there would be no mix-up later in whose baby belong to whom.

Because we had many tiny people in the nursery, and not a lot of extra staff on hand, we used a special conveyance to get them out for their feedings. Taking the baby's out to their mothers one at a time took too long, and when a baby was hungry it let us know, loudly, it wanted to be fed. It was imperative, therefore for everyone's wellbeing, that we deliver our tiny charges to their respective mothers without any delay.

On this particular maternity ward we had a special vehicle which we could use to take out a large number of babies all at the same time. It was like an oversized stretcher with crib-style slots that kept each baby separate from its next door neighbor.

The routine was that every infant's surname was written on a piece of soft paper, which was then put in a groove. The baby was weighed, changed and name verified, before being bunny wrapped and placed into its respective area. Once the cart was full, of usually crying babies, the nurse would proceed to deliver them to their rightful owners.

If we were extra busy, we would sometimes tuck another infant under an arm, while at the same time pushing the cart down the hall with the free hand. Maybe it was not a perfect method but it seemed to be an efficient time saving technique for both the babies and the nursery staff.

Now here was this mother telling me that I'd made a ghastly mistake, and that the baby that I had thought was hers, wasn't. I felt sick. If this were my fault and I had got the babies mixed up the consequences for me would not be good. I knew that the Director of Nursing did not condone incompetence of any kind.

In the nursery I'd been so certain I had got everything right. I stood struggling to think of how I could have made such a horrible blunder.

The four women watched me as I tried to collect my thoughts. I took a minute to look at the babe resting in my arms and then at the mother who was holding out her arms to receive it. I looked closely again at the small face and back to the woman in the bed. No way, I thought, this couldn't be right. The mother did not look anything, as the baby she said was hers.

Just at that moment the first woman roared with laugher, and that is when I cottoned on that something was going on that involved me. I stood at the end of the second mum's bed still clutching the small bundle. By this time all four occupants of that room were consumed in gales of laughter.

"Oh! Nurse, " the first mother giggled. "You should have seen your face when I told you that baby wasn't mine. It went white and you started to bite your bottom lip."

She broke again into peals of merriment and the others joined in. I was not amused by what was happening. It was a nasty shock.

I still had a number of hungry babies to deliver, and more waiting for me. My peers would also be wondering where I was and why I was taking so long.

Placing the baby on the end of the first mother's bed, I removed his blanket. I looked at the name on his back. Then I checked the lady's armband to see if their names matched. With relief I discovered that they were the same. I quickly bundled up her baby and swiftly handed him over to her.

She looked slightly embarrassed as she took him. " I didn't mean any harm by it you know. We were just having a wee bit of fun with you, that is all." The other three mothers nodded.

The first perpetrator frowned, and peered anxiously at me. "I hope you're not going to report us or anything like that?"

I was provoked by all the time that we had wasted by this foolish prank. I did not trust myself to speak so I shook my head.

As fast as I could, and without making any further conversation, I gave the other mothers their infants. As I hurried back to collect my other small charges, I could still hear those four women giggling aloud.

From that day, however, I never again handed over a baby before checking its name against the name-band of its mother. It took a bit longer to do this but it was my way of making certain that there was not another such incident.

Unquestionable Acceptance

"Don't fuss so nurse, I'm fine- really I am." The elderly woman said, smiling at me.

Gladys Stevens was in her early nineties. She had come to our ward because of a chronic heart condition. The plan was to try and get her stabilized and then hopefully send her back home. This was to be done by removing some of the build up of fluid around her heart as well as improving her medications.

As happens so many times this one did not work out as the medical team hoped. However, it taught me another lesson; never underestimate the inner strengths that people possess.

"Nurse," Gladys well lined, small face peeked out from under the pile of bedclothes. "Nurse I'm alright, and I'd really like to take a nap." She popped a hand out and patted my arm. Please, don't fret about me anymore, even though it's much appreciated." Her kindly face smiled.

"Well, if you're quite sure you are comfortable........I'll go." Gladys had closed her eyes. I just made sure she could reach her call bell before exiting her room.

This woman was an avid knitter. She told me that over the years she must have knitted hundreds of pairs of mitts for mission services.

"I like to do them, "she had told me on many occasions, because they came together quickly." According to her, no one would needlessly suffer with cold hands in the winter as long as she was able to knit."

Later returning to her room, I found her awake and trying to sit up on the edge of her bed. Alright," I said, taking a firm hold of her, "and, just what do you think you're doing?"

"I thought I'd see if I could get myself up. I didn't plan on doing anything too strenuous, but..."She sighed. "I've found out that's even getting too much for these old bones.

Pulling the oxygen cord free from the hook on the wall I placed the prongs into her nose and switched it on. "You lie back down Gladys, while you get a little of help with your air intake.

After her breathing had become easier, I helped her to sit up again on the edge of the bed. "Now, would you like to sit in your chair?"

"Yes please nurse. Perhaps I can do a little bit of my needlework." We slowly eased her frail body into a chair.

As I was getting her comfortable one of Gladys daughters arrived. Dorothy came frequently to see her mother so she was a familiar sight on the ward. She came over to her mother and gently kissed her on the forehead.

"You're looking a lot better today." Dorothy beamed. "That's really great Mum."

Gladys smiled. "Yes, I'm feeling not too bad today. Which is a nice change."

"Yes, your mum is better today," I said looking at Dorothy, "but when she gets short of breath she needs to wear her oxygen. She doesn't like to do that but it is for the best."

Mrs. Stevens's daughter had removed her coat, and sat down beside her mother. "Did you hear that, mother?" she scolded.

"Oh my goodness, yes, I heard what my nurse said." Gladys nodded. "But, what difference does it make? I know I'm dying and..."

"Mum, please stop that." Dorothy said, her voice trembling. "You are not dying." She looked over at me. "Please, nurse, will you tell her that she is not going to die."

The anguish in Dorothy's voice was intense. I would have loved to repeat what she had said, but I knew down deeply that what my patient had uttered at was closer to the truth.

"My dear girl," Gladys took hold of her daughter's hands, " look at me. I am an old tired lady. I'm not afraid of dying."

She stroked the hand nestled in her own. "This nurse knows how I feel about death, I've spoken to her about this many times."

Dorothy looked quizzical at me. "She's talked with you concerning this?"

"Yes, " I said. "We have talked often about life, and she has spoken about her own strong beliefs." I looked into this middle-aged woman's sad face. "Your mother is a unique lady."

"I know that. I know that." Dorothy sobbed. "And, it hurts me so to hear her talking about dying, "

"I'm sure it must be very painful for you to think about your mother's life ending. It is never an easy thing to accept. If you would like to talk with someone else about this I can arrange that for you."

Dorothy shook her head. "No, that won't be necessary but thank you anyway."

Gladys smiled, as she raised her daughter's hand to her lips and kissed it.

"My daughter knows I've always believed that death is but another phase to life. It holds no fear at all for me."

"Oh! Mum please don't" Dorothy implored.

Mrs. Stevens looked lovingly at her daughter. "I've got to talk about it because I know that any time I have left is short. Please dear, " again she kissed her daughters hand, "promise me, that when it's my time you'll let me go."

This was becoming a delicate issue. As I had other work to do, I thought it best if I left them alone.

When I returned to her room I found Gladys sitting up in bed reading her Bible. I always found that when a patient held a strong belief that there was life after death, it helped them embrace it better and made the nurse's role a little easier.

"Your daughter got away alright Gladys?" I said.

She smiled and nodded.

"Yes, and would you believe we even spoke about the kind of memorial service I'd like. Dorothy has always been the stronger of my two daughters. What is hard for her is that we have also always been close.

I smiled, and glanced at the passage she was reading. It was from the book of Psalms.

"That's one of my favorite books of the Bible, " I said.

"It's a best loved one of mine too, " Gladys beamed. "It really says it all. We do not have anything to fear. Have faith and believe."

I saw she was reading the 23rd psalm, and as I knew the words, I nodded in agreement. "Even though I walk through the valley of the shadow of death; I fear no evil; for thou art with me."

"Yes." I said. "I do believe those words can be very comforting. Also, I am pleased that you and your daughter were able to be more open with each other."

"Well, nurse, as I've told her I do not want a mournful memorial service. Instead, I have asked her to promise me that she will see that it is more a celebration of my life. I've lived a long life and I've been a most fortunate lady in numerous ways."

She sighed. "I have just got to convince my daughter of this. That when we die its simply another door which we go through to something more grander than we can imagine.""

I leant over and gave her a hug. She hugged me back.

"You know, nurse, meeting you has been a lovely experience."

"Well it's been super for me, Mrs. Stevens as well. Now let's fix your covers. I think you deserve to take a little rest before your supper arrives."

"Yes that sounds nice, " she said, snuggling down under the blankets. Just leave my Bible nearby."

Gladys suffered through the procedure to remove the excess fluid from around her heart. After that her condition deteriorated, but she never once protested. Her total acceptance of what was happening is something I'll remember about her.

Following her mother's funeral Dorothy sent me a copy of one of the readings from the service. The piece is entitled Miss Me - But Let Me Go, author unknown. The first verse says, " When I come to the end of the road, and the sun has set for me, I want no rites in a gloom filled room, Why cry for a soul set free.

Those words for me completely summed up how Gladys wanted her family to look at her passing. The fact that they were able to finally do that I'm sure pleased her as much as it did me.

Will Power can be Amazing

Gladys blue beady eyes glared at me over the top of the bedclothes. She held them tightly up around her small pointed chin.

"Just get out of my room and leave me alone, " she snarled at us. " I want to have a sleep. Can't you see I'm a sick old woman."

I smiled at Ray, my co-worker. I had asked him to help get Gladys up for a walk. " Well what do you think.? Should we make her get out of her bed?" I
frowned, thinking that this wasn't going to be easy. It was obvious from her body language my patient didn't want to go anywhere.

"The doctors have ordered an increase in Mrs. Barton's activities, " I added. " I'm supposed to get her out walking in the halls, at least a couple of times a day."

Ray looked at me with raised eyebrows and grinned. " I don't think you are going to get very far today walking this lady. Perhaps we could just sit her on the side of the bed. That at least would be a start."

I attempted to get the covers off Gladys. A thin arm shot out from under them. She tried to grab hold of my hand but I quickly backed out of her reach.

"Get out of here, she yelled. "Leave me alone. I'm not well and none of you care."

"Gladys, it's because we do care about you that we want to help you get stronger."

I leant over her and tried to make eye contact. She immediately scrunched her eyes shut.

Ray smiled. " Well, I don't know about you but I've got lots of my own work to do. If you want to try again later just come and get me." He waved as he left the room.

"Now do you see what you've done Mrs. Barton." There was no movement from the bed. Gladys still had a firm grasp of the covers and her eyes remained clamped shut.

"I'm going to leave you for a little while." I said. "But I'll be back." Gladys eyes flickered for a moment and a cheeky grin flashed across her small features.

"The next time Mrs. Barton," I spoke close to her ear, "you are going to get up and you will go for a walk just as the doctors have ordered."

This elderly lady had come to our floor from a nursing home. In her mid-eighties, she had needed an assessment of her emphysema, a chronic breathing problem. She was now much improved and the medical team wanted to discharge her, but first we needed to get her mobile. It was obvious from her behavior she wasn't going to be a willing participant in this venture.

Later that same day I cornered Ray, and again we headed back into Gladys room. She was sitting on the commode, which she had by her bedside.

When she saw us she made a mad scramble trying to get off it and get back into bed. Nevertheless, I took hold of one of her arms and Ray held onto the other so she was not able to go anywhere.

"Let go of me, " she spat at us. " I'm telling you right now if you don't help me back into my bed, I'll....I'll see you both lose your jobs as nurses."

Gladys squirmed and wriggled as she yelled. Ray and I had a firm hold of her, even when we stood her up to attend to her personal needs, so she was not able to get free.

"I'm not going anywhere, so you can just put me right back in my bed." She demanded.

"Okay that's just about enough of that, Mrs. Barton, " I said, " Look at you. You're standing up fine. You are not the least bit

180

wobbly on your feet, and I've been ordered to get you out walking in the hall."

Ray and I had now had her positioned ready to walk. "Let's go Gladys." I told her firmly.

This elderly woman flatly refused to move her feet. When we moved her away from her bed, she hung between us as a limp doll, with her slippers dragging across the floor.

Ray gave a loud laughed. " Oh! Brother is this ever one stubborn lady. She's got a will all of her own."

"Well that's good, " I retorted, "because she's going to see that I can be just as obstinate as she is."

"Help! Help! They are trying to kill me." Gladys screamed as we slowly made our way down the hall. She still wouldn't walk so we continued to pull her along making sure that she was in no danger of being injured.

"Gladys you are really being very silly, " I said, "you know that you're well enough to be discharged so you're just belaboring what's unavoidable. Why?"

Gladys muttered something crossly under her breath. I wasn't able to make it out.

"What did you say?" I asked her.

"I don't want to go back to that place."

"Well I'm sorry you feel that way but this is a hospital not a long term care facility."

Ray looked across at me. "Okay, enough of this. Let's take Mrs. Barton back to her room. This isn't working. You'll need to inform the team of that, maybe they can suggest something else."

To turn Gladys we had both released our hold of her. She immediately took off leaving Ray and I standing watching her departure with utter astonishment.

We both laughed at how fast Gladys had moved. It was obvious from her agility she had no problems at all getting around.

When I walked back into Gladys room, I found her back in her bed. Her eyes shut tight and her body completely covered with blankets. I could see she was comfortable so I left her alone.

Gladys continued to play up whenever we attempted to get her walking, but every time we turned to go back to her room she always beat us to it. The speed she was able to muster to do this was incredible for someone of her age.

Once the medical team was informed of Mrs. Bartons' ability to move quicker than most of us, she was discharged. Even though Gladys was an elderly, frail looking lady she was living proof that size and age count for little against sheer stubbornness and a strong will power. Remembering those particular attributes of this lady, and even though many years have past, they still make me smile.